TOGETHER BEHIND FOUR WALLS

A COLLECTION OF IMAGES, SHORT STORIES AND POEMS SUPPORTING MARIE CURIE NURSES

Compiled by
Francis H Powell

Graphic design: Dena Villanueva

A CIP catalogue record of this book is available from the British Library.

Published by Goldcrest Books International Ltd
www.goldcrestbooks.com
publish@goldcrestbooks.com

ISBN: 978-1-913719-34-0

CONTENTS

I

INTRODUCTION

On a cold grey March morning, I was with my son, in the play park where he regularly plays, when all of a sudden some council workers began cordoning off the play park. He was not able to go to school, due to a sudden outbreak of covid 19 cases in the local area. The closing off of the play area really brought home the fact that something significant was beginning to impact our lives and the normal life we were used to was about to change dramatically. Consequently, I began to put words to my feelings at the time and all of a sudden the idea of putting a book together, came to me. I began rifling through my contacts and friends who were writers. Later I began to search further afield, sending e mails to people explaining my project. I knew I wanted to put a book together for those who would be caring for people, doing valuable work, such as nurses and by way of my sister I, decided Marie Curie Nurses were a good cause, who should benefit from this fund-raising project. I am grateful to all those who responded to my call for poems, short stories and illustrations, as well as people who have helped to publicize this project. I am incredibly fortunate some fantastic writers and poets, who at the onset I could never imagine would

submit poems, kindly sent me some pertinent works. I like the range of writers and poets who have contributed to this book, from a ninety-one year old writer, poet Lynne Reid Banks, who is obviously still passionate about writing to young children.
I would also like to dedicate this book to two much missed family members, firstly Johnnie Maclean, who was looked after by Marie Curie Nurses, as well as my oldest sister, Elizabeth Harden, who I feel certain would have been out and about helping people during the covid 19 crisis. This book is a chronicle to a terrible global crisis in which many people lost their loved ones and many were forced into an unanticipated lock down. A special thanks to Dena Villanuava for the graphics work. Giselle Marks for the editing. Sarah J Waldock for the initial formatting of the book.

Francis H Powell

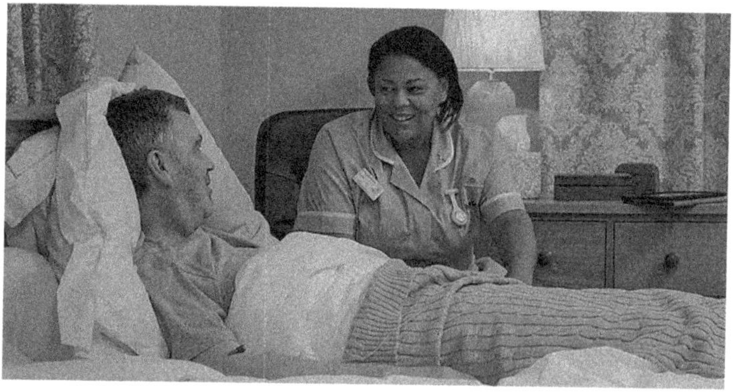

MARIE CURIE NURSES

Marie Curie nurses in our communities and hospices provide hands on nursing care to patients at the end of their lives. Throughout the Corona Virus Pandemic, our nurses have been at the frontline of care, looking after patients with all terminal illnesses, including caring for people with the virus.

The need for our work has never been greater. At the time when our nurses are in such demand, we have also faced a devastating loss in our income.

When living with a terminal illness it is vital that you can access crucial support, care and information. Your support in buying this book, is enabling our frontline staff to continue to provide that expert care along with the vital bereavement advice and guidance we also provide to carers and families having to deal with loss and grief.

CARING AND KINDNESS

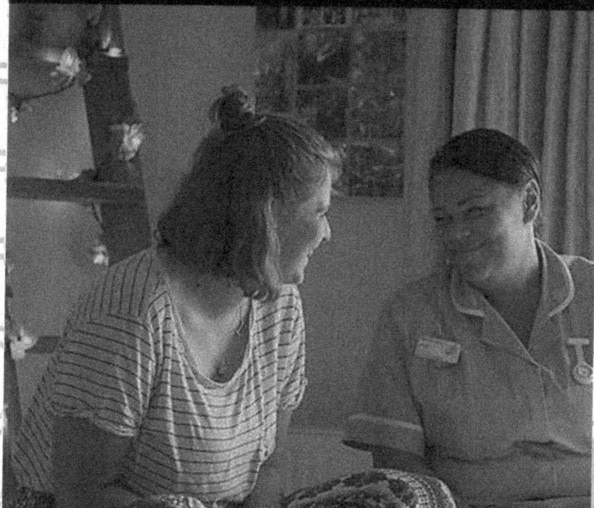

Roger Robinson, John Hegley, Arthur Smith,
Francis H Powell, Tavinder Kaur New,
P.J.Reed Magi Gibson, Tom Stockley,
Laura Mucha, ChrissieGittens

Grace

Roger Robinson

That year we danced to green bleeps on screen.
My son had come early, just the 1kg of him,
all big head, bulging eyes and blue veins.

On the ward I met Grace. A Jamaican senior nurse
who sang pop songs on her shift, like they were hymns.
"Your son feisty. Y'see him just ah pull off the breathing mask."

People spoke of her in half tones down these carbolic halls.
Even the doctors gave way to her, when it comes
to putting a line into my son's nylon thread of a vein.

She'd warn junior doctors with trembling hands: "Me only
letting you try twice."

On her night shift she pulls my son's incubator into her room,
no matter the tangled confusion of wires and machine.

When the consultant told my wife and I on morning rounds
that he's not sure my son will live, and if he lives he might never
leave the hospital, she pulled us quickly aside: "Him have no
right to say that just raw so."

Another consultant tells the nurses to stop feeding a baby,
who will soon die,
and she commands her loyal nurses to feed him. "No baby
must dead wid a hungry belly." And she'd sit in the dark,
rocking that well-fed baby,

held to her bosom, slowly humming the melody of "Happy"
by Pharrell.

And I think, if by some chance, I'm not here and my son's life
should flicker, then Grace, she should be the one

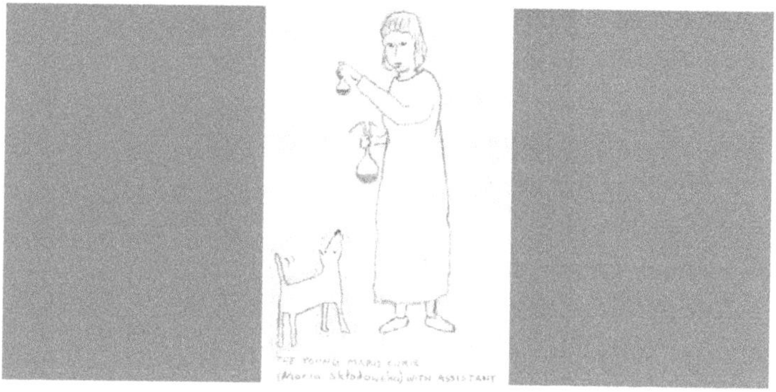

Marie Curie

John Hegley

Marie Curie - isolated
when her work began:
a scientific world
made more for man and boy than woman.
But, Marie Curie she became
a winner of the Nobel prize
and Albert Einstein said
she was,
'the only one who fame has not corrupted.'

Marie Curie, she was married
in a dress of blue,
the same one she wore in the lab
with Pierre, her husband who
helped isolate the radium
which Marie Curie found
would undo the sickly cells
more quickly than the healthy ones around them.

She founded radiation units
in the First World War.
She tried to sell her Nobel medals
to help the effort more.
She carried in her white coat pocket,
occasionally, a phial
of radium -for it would be a while
before the knowledge of the danger.
So, even now, there's things of hers,
kept in a box of lead.

Marie Curie, born in Warsaw,
Paris - worked and wed.
Marie Curie, pure of fury,
heart and soul and head.

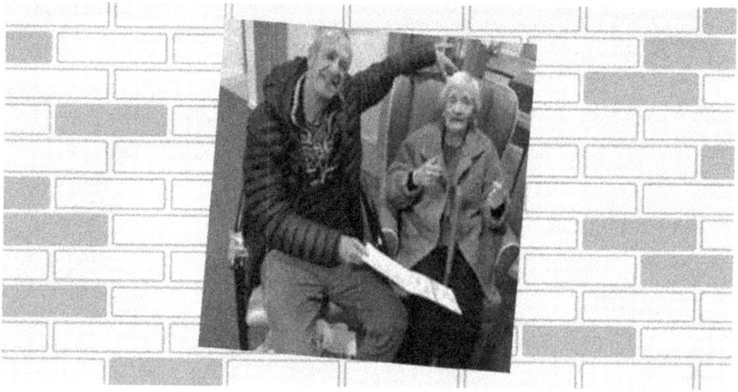

May 8th 2020

Arthur Smith

Oh mother, I cannot see you today
though I know you are bathed
in the tender warmth
of those who care for you.
And I know too
that as your head rocks gently
among hidden rhythms
that there she still is,
the grammar school girl
from Camberwell Green,
laughing among friends
in the whirling blossoms
of relief and hope,
dancing, kissing sailors
in Trafalgar Square.
It is VE day
and the rest of the century
is yours.

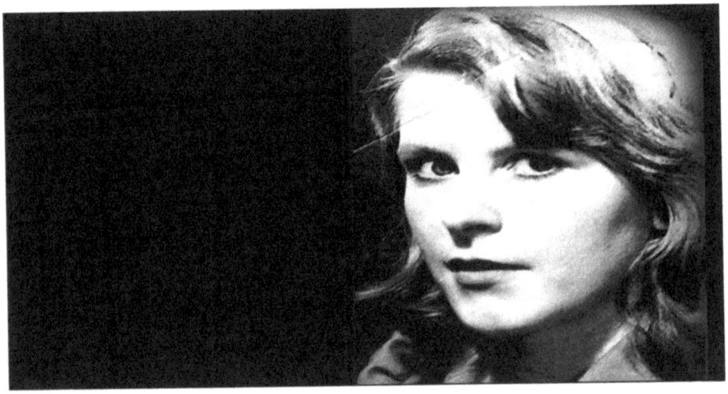

A Tribute

Francis H Powell

My sister would have been out there
I know she would
delivering food parcels
doing as much as she could
She would have been there
of that I am sure
making a difference
from door to door

A year has passed
but her spirit lives on
she would have been out there
because she cared
salutations from her heart
with her soul laid bare
A wrap on the door
an accompanied smile

an affinity with people
always offering her time
an unquenchable interest
in other people's lives
like an old gypsy
she once she cared for
whose story tickled her mind

She was once a nurse
in a lifetime of giving
going about her life
with a hunger to please
If you had ever met her
you would know
what I mean
Her heart worn openly
displayed on her sleeve
An element of my world
is missing by her absence
She would always be there
in anyone's moment of need
She would have taken the world's burden
right in her arms
an abiding faith and hope
was part of her charms

She would have been there
in the thick of it all
doing whatever was needed
to make a difference
putting herself on the line
a rose amongst brambles and thorns.

Then and Now

Tavinder Kaur New

Rushing, dashing, getting up early to get to work that was then,
Sitting at home, resting, relaxing watching Netflix that is now,

All we have been asked to do is sit indoors and save the NHS,

In the past, people were asked to go to war, work in the factors,
All we have been asked to do is sit indoors and save the NHS
We have internet, What'sApp, YouTube and the internet
this is now,
In the past all they had were the radio, letters and black and
white TV

All we have been asked to do is sit indoors and save the NHS.

We will see our families, colleagues and friends again when this
is over
In the past COVID 19 will be a distance memory and lives will
be saved

So stay indoors, stay apart, save lives and the NHS!

On the Hospice End of Life Ward

Magi Gibson

There's a window in the slanting roof
above the beds where the patients lie.

The sky flits slowly past; a gallery
of ever-changing photographs.

Watch as a perfect sheet of blue
shifts to a blur of stormy tears.

Doze off to a blank of boring grey,
wake to a silver moon as it ghostly

trails thin veils of cloud across the dark.
Some say that on windless nights

when the sky is clear and deep,
you might even see heaven,

and drifting off to sleep, might hear
the voices of angels speak

softly, by the nurses' station.

Careworker

Tom Stockley

I have had a lot of time, recently, to think about things
which is definitely what a closet introvert needs.
i've been thinking about how i've been taught to care
 for people
but always skipped the lessons about looking after myself.
i've been seeing people sweeping driveways,
planting seeds
and learning to be human again
and my capacity for love is somehow greater than it's ever
 been before
so much so that, maybe,
i might have some left for myself.

Dear Key Workers

Laura Mucha in collaboration with children around the world during the coronavirus pandemic in 2020

You sprint, lift and listen
to heartbeats, worries,
and the puff
    and gasp
of ventilators.
You inject painkillers
    and courage.

You teach history,
    hockey
        and hope.
You grow
    imaginations
        confidence,
    brains.
You believe in us,
    you care.

You soak, scrub
    and sweep
        away our fears.
You put out fires
    and warm our spirits.
You bring letters,
    lifelines,
    and love.

You pick, pack, stack,
    prepare.
You keep shelves
    and bellies full.
You nourish us.
    You share.

You govern, guide, inform,
    protect,
search, rescue, build,
    arrest.
You comfort.
    You mend.

You keep our streets clean,
    and our minds tidy.
No matter what, you're there.

Super People

Chrissie Gittens

(Captain Tom spoke on BBCR4 about the 'super people' who support his campaign to raise funds for N.H.S. Charities Together)

Super people wear masks and bandanas,
Super people run around the park and sometimes make eye contact,
Super people are spoken to the police because they've been seen
leaving their house more than once a day.

Super people leave their house more than once a day because they shop
for the housebound and volunteer at the food bank,
Super people don't wear masks and bandanas,
Super people phone their friends while they are sitting outside
and have no idea of the time.

Super people forget if they've washed their hands so they wash them again,
Super people get on with planting seeds and are continually aghast when
a bean stem rises like a lollipop,
Super people get on with soundproofing their flat for they are expecting
a baby in July and don't want to disturb their neighbours.

Super people remember to water their plants,
Super people walk round the park, smile and say, 'Good Morning',

Super people offer to add your food items to their Tesco
  delivery slot.

Super people pile their front windows with paper
  Easter eggs
including one with a rainbow,
Super people don't tell their children it's the Easter holidays
to avoid breaking their routine,
Super people say 'Take your time' when they deliver a
humungous amount of shopping to your doorstep.

Super people don't get ill,
Super people don't get ill,
Super people do get ill,
Super people watch the new leaves hurtling from one tree
  to another.

Twenty-Twenty Fashion

P.J. Reed

Furloughed families
in daytime pyjamas,
support the NHS.
Stay-at-home heroes
draw rainbows and clap,
bang on saucepan lids
while social distancing
among manicured gardens,
in little family bubbles and
annoy the night-time workers.

They listen to daily briefings
watch 'R' rate rise and fall
in this pandemic waltz.
Scurrying to the open shops
in homemade PPE.
Old floral sheets and
ugly, unused scarves
wrapped tightly around
sweating faces
and fogging glasses,
in twenty-twenty fashion.

DEEP THOUGHTS

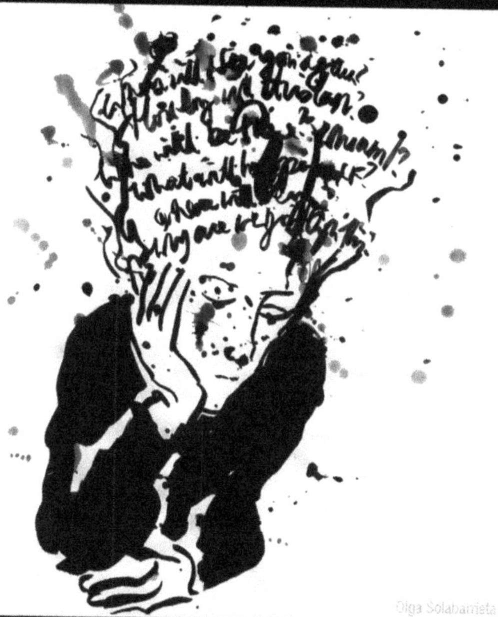

Olga Solabarrieta

By the Poet, Bruno de Oliveira, Barnabas Wetton, Virna Teixera, David Field, Josiane Vincent, Nobert Gora, Stéphanie Hulbert-Powell, Wendy Cope OBE, Arti Rai, Leela Soma, Sarah J. Waldock, Serena Braida, Toby Campion, Giselle Marks, Dylan Tynan, Tom Stockley, Nicholas McGaughey, Margot Henderson, Hadley-James Hoyles, Muni Subhradip Chakraborty, Tim Turnbull, Martin Figura, Alison Brakenbury, Graham Clifford, Paul Isolani Smyth, Andrena Zawinski, David K McDonald, Okorie Harrison

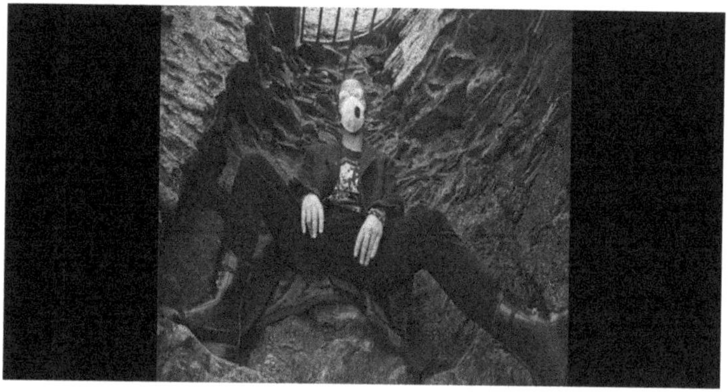

Love the Void

B the Poet

If you should dissipate,
Please take me with you,
I vow to hereby love the void.
I pledge my alliance to the hopeless,
I offer my soul to nothing at all.
If you should dissipate,
Please take me with you,
Scatter shatter letters,
Leave me a trail of lost lexis,
If you dissipate,
Before you go,
Feed me a story,
For I feel hollow,
Plant me a garden,
Within the emptiness of my ribcage,
If you should dissipate,

Leave me your voice,
Cotton soft,
And although you have gone,
I still hear your sway.
If you should dissipate,
Leave me your legacy.

A New Horizon

Bruno de Oliveira

What we are experiencing today will go down in history as the greatest demonstration for resilience, solidarity and a fellow-spirit in the history of our generation.

For forty years, we have grown far apart. We question as if there were not such a thing as society. Through this moment of crisis, we have found humanity once lost where I am my neighbour's support and help. If my neighbour can't go to the shop to feed herself, it is my problem. If my neighbour can't get to a hospital, it is my problem. If my neighbour can't pay his rent, it is my problem. In a time of crisis, a new hope is born where we no longer see ourselves as a competitor, but as a collaborator. Science has pointed to the value of synergism.

We must see that together there is a new horizon in front of us. We will overcome this crisis, and we will be able to hold the hands of each other again. But, we must see that, on the horizon, our neighbours, our friends and our family should not have to struggle to feed themselves, worry about having a roof above their heads, or about having to pay to receive medical care. May this time unite us as we regain pleasure inhearing the birds singing.

We are on this planet truly together. From policy makers to the delivery drivers, from the nurse to the shopkeepers, from a new-born baby to the centenarian. There is an air that unifies us. The sound of our hands that we momentarily can no longer hold, still brings us joy as it comes together in the form of clapping to end the temporary isolation. Our hands are still bringing us together. We build a sound of humanity, of our fellowship as humans.

Through our windows, a light of hope is framed by this shared moment. In a sense, we have been reunited, and as mother history taught us, we must forge new and stronger bonds. In this unfathomable universe, we only have each other. We will come out of this dark tunnel. We will, and we must use the dim light that shines in front of us to establish a new contract for the blessing of humankind - a more equitable and equal society. A new rainbow of equals for a more united world.

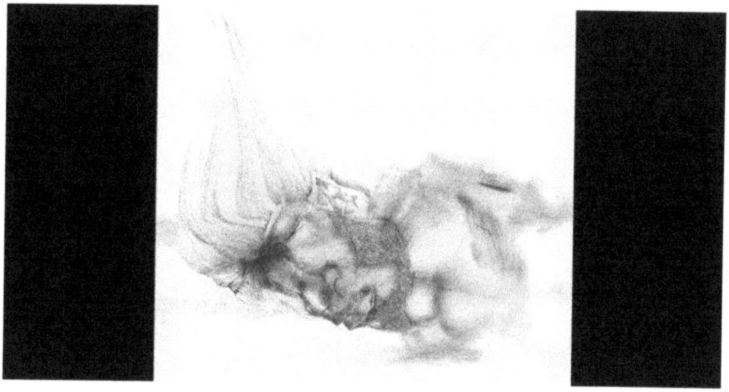

To Bath Alone

Barnabas Wetton

Each of our homes is
wrapped in the insolence
of tasks badly done
and the same re-found lists
run over again and re-run

In this time of shadows and light
we are all bathing alone,
wet from the memory of before
and dry to any hope of tomorrow.

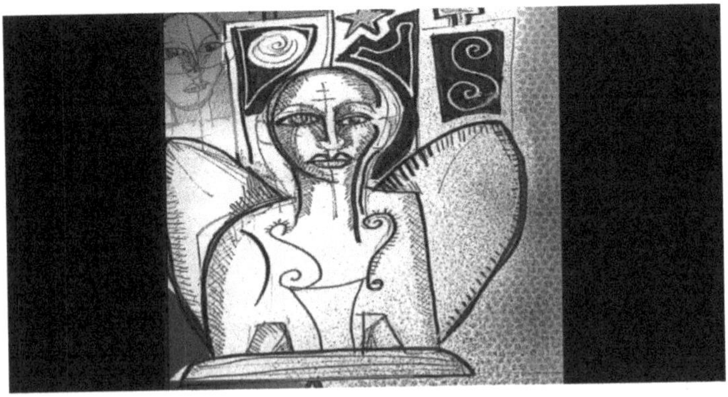

Between Losses and Miracles

Virna Teixera

I didn't write for a few days because although I got better, I had to deal with difficult circumstances linked to Covid-19, including the loss of a person dear to me who had a severe form of the disease. I followed the whole process closely, from the onset of symptoms to his admission to the hospital, and the two weeks he spent in the ICU. His hypoxia-confused messages on WhatsApp before incubation. His request that 'Virna the medic' take care of communication with the medical team. The family's anguish every day, his wife who was isolated at home, recovering.

Contact with the hospital is by telephone only. The ICU number is always busy or no one answers. Information is usually provided through the nursing staff. So you wait twenty-four hours to hear a "stable on the respirator" or something. Or an excess of medical details that make the family uneasy. I have never felt so helpless as a doctor from afar, and I know that the feeling of helplessness is universal right now among healthcare professionals. However, a few times I had to make myself heard, and demanded more precise information directly from a colleague. Even in communication there are echoes of isolation. I feel sorry for the people who are currently hospitalized, and for those who are dealing with hard losses caused by this horrendous virus. There is the dark side of respirators too, and the aftermath of recovery. It is not just about miraculously surviving an ICU.

I listen skeptically to hydroxychloroquine enthusiasts, especially my Brazilian colleagues. Some of them, by the way, are enthusiastic theoreticians in specialties far from the front. Some of them are isolated in their apartments, scared to death of contracting the virus. The British do not use hydroxychloroquine. They are right. There is no evidence. The CDC, embarrassed, removed Trump's hard-hitting drug from the recommendations on its website.

It is not that I am against attempts, but I do not see much scientific method in this "miracle". What I see is a tiny amount of research undertaken with debatable methodology, and anecdotal reports shared in hospital corridors and last-minute training classes. We have taken it easy, and we know that in Brazil and elsewhere there are mainly political interests behind this move. The number of infections and deaths continues to rise at an alarming rate worldwide. There are other research medications against viral replication that look more promising. I think that suddenly one could try to use Ayahuasca for Covid-19 in Brazil. I don't know why, but I have more faith in Ayahuasca than hydroxychloroquine. It must be my Brazilian spiritualist side.

Maybe I became cynical after watching Zoom's first online funeral, which was absolutely surreal. It is a kind of support, but until recently it was something unimaginable. Anyway, I no longer have patience with boring people who come to you with their lying pseudo-compassion, to talk about themselves, their little histrionic dramas. I also have zero tolerance for cowardly 'covidiots' locked up in their homes with imaginary, narcissistic symptoms, sharing articles as stupid as they are, these ridiculous articles they read in the media, and thinking themselves to be authorities on the subject. A little alcohol gel in the cerebral cortex would do them a world of good. And I cheer for those who have made more productive and creative decisions in their lives at this time, despite the crisis.

About the close person who died. He was an extraordinary and generous man. He had a beautiful life. He was 75 years old, and an athlete. He fought bravely on the respirator, but his time came. Death is also part of life. It's been over fifteen days since I got the virus and I'm almost healed. My senses of taste and smell returned. I'm alive. My mood has lifted. I cooked a beautiful meal, drank half a bottle of wine, and listened to old songs, my way of dealing with the loss of a wonderful man who knew how to live and enjoyed the good things in life. I thought of the famous excerpt from Shakespeare's Julius Caesar, 'a coward dies a thousand times before his death, but the valiant taste death but once'.

Translated by Chris Daniels

Fire and Water

David Field

Rumi said, more elegantly than this,
that when we are young,
and see fire
on our path,
we dive into water to avoid it.

But when older,
if we have learned anything at all,
and see fire
on our path,
we walk into it.

Water is for later.

You have known fire.
You have known water.

And to my eye,
you step calmly into fire,
and when it is time for water...
otters...
smile to see you.

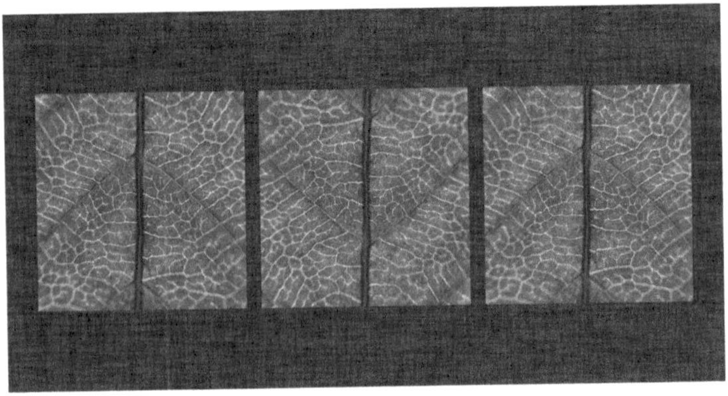

If you Were

Josiane Vincent

IF YOU WERE
Tell me
How would you fancy your surroundings
If you were...

If I were a painter
I would paint a still life
A la Pollock though
Drops dripping
Splashes smashing
On a large canvas
At random
A mute landscape
springing out of nowhere
Metaphorical show of
Baffled colours
Telling the metaphysics of

A city gone to sleep
A colourless spell has
cleared out the boulevard

If I were a film maker
I would shoot a silent film
Filling the screen
A speeded-up motion of
A crowd of people
Bursting about
A flock of pigeons
Flying off
The hubbub of city life
Deaf and dumb
The oracle is still in the limbo
When out of the blue
The momentum slowing down
The impetus of life
anaesthesized
A clamour arises
In the dark(ness)
Blurred visions of
Still snapshots
On and off
On and off
Until
A fine ribbon
Stretches out
As far as the eyes can see
Void is the boulevard
Asleep is the city

Life We Used to Live

Nobert Gora

Droplets fall on the floor,
they multiply like during a rainy act,
but this isn't a manifestation of Mother Earth,
it's the nature of an exhausted man.

These are tears of powerlessness
which blur the old world
and cover fresh memories of normality
(now everyone needs them like oxygen).

Distance between people,
mass-media spit out fear,
it all doesn't look like life,
life we used to live.

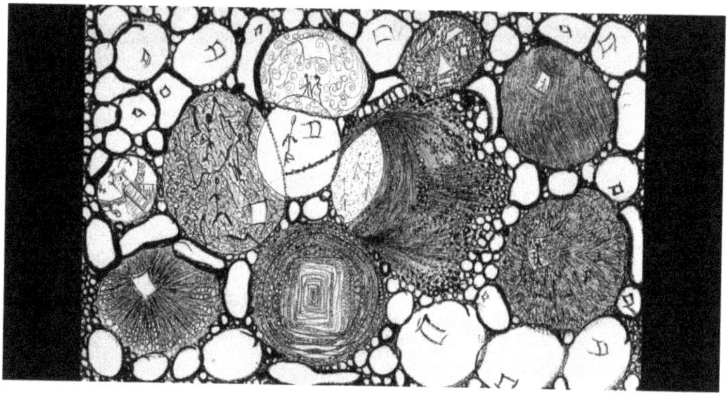

Locked In

Stéphanie Hulbert-Powell

Blue is the sky
Empty are the streets
Full is my head with thoughts,
Darkened by the news in the world.
Sit silently, try to let go,
Drowned in memories of a time that is no more.
Be aware and don't follow the rising reflection
Fighting against rumination,
Entrapped again
Feeling powerless, facing the limits within.
Faraway fear approaching
End of the day
Try to remember its ending development.

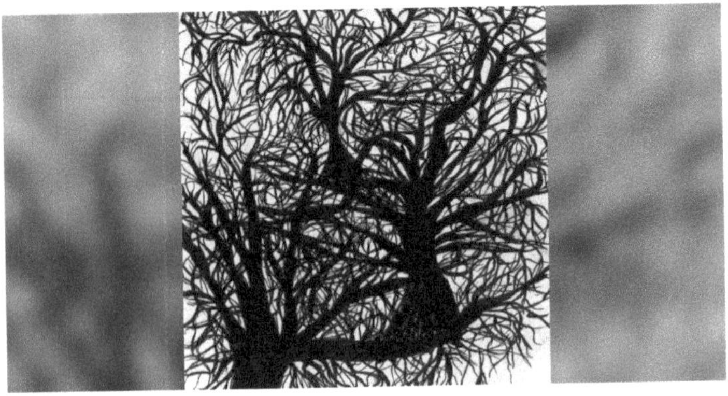

Naga Uta

Wendy Cope OBE

Now I can't walk far
I head to the nearest park
where seventeen trees
are my enchanted forest.
In their dappled shade.
I breathe slowly, touch the bark.
Somewhere a bird is singing.

(*Naga uta* is a Japanese form)

Never

Arti Rai

A single candle flickering,
fighting for its breaths,
struggling tough when life
is dead eclipsed all over,
holds divinity and faith
all against despondance,
kindles a ray of life
In the sky of murkiness.
What's bad if I hold one
and pledge –
"I won't surrender even when
the God of Hell is all powerful.
I'm life, I won't give up ever
NEVER."

Pen

Leela Soma

"The Pen is the tongue of the mind." Miguel de Cervantes
The letters of the alphabets fuse in colour in
a black and white landscape of wounds and pain
Words I wish to use, as naked as I want them to be
in these strange times of the pandemic.

Voices float from the television, gowns, PPE,
gloves, random numbers creep up every day,
the incredible daily toll of infections, deaths, in graphs,
as families behind those figures, mourn their loved ones,
words become silent.

I circle the days in the Covid-19 diary, add words,
a shrine of words, on a blank page, bury feelings
time passes like the still waters of the pond
a hush, then a flow as I untie the bond of words.

Ordinary events of birth, marriage, illness, old age
and death have a new meaning in this silent world
Outside the window birds' chirp, leaves dance in the wind, sun
shines, would I be able to breathe life into words?

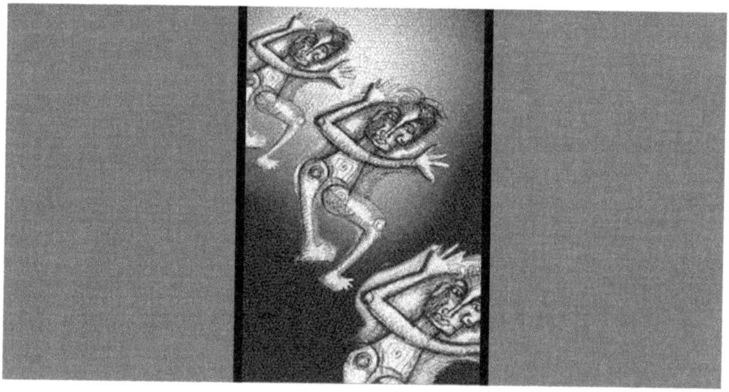

Sapphic Ode to Corona Virus19

Sarah J. Waldock

Corona virus sneaks unseen, unheard
Passing with cough or sneeze, or spat out word
To coyly creep into each new host's lung
A tale unsung

The virus minions lurk in places warm
Like unwashed hands; infected faces swarm
The myriad germs in army ranks to go
Assault their foe

They colonise the host and with much glee
Use stolen DNA asexually
To reproduce and, ready for the fray
Get coughed away

Beware the careless meetings, friendly kiss
Beware the unmasked night of casual bliss!
The pox, and AIDS, Clamydia close your eyes
At CoV's rise!

Sheila's Speech

Serena Braida

sometimes things stick to me

like I am a wall
like I am the firmament

and the cold elastic joy
of the drugged tongue

sometimes they stick to me
krystal and blue

kilos, sometimes, a crack
in the door

St Teresa flexed
loud and light

First published in *Blue Sheila*, Dancing Girl Press (Chicago, 2018)

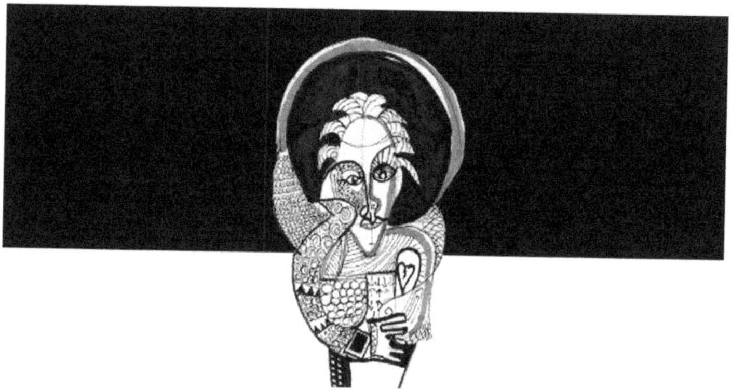

Service Note to Self

Toby Campion (U.S.)

Who's trending now? Who's hot?
My selfie self is not.
My Facebook friends are ailing,
my server feed is failing.

If God could text me now—
just one emoji, wow!
From yottabytes, A Face,
streaming gladness, grace.

Just joking, cyber moles,
you memer geeks and trolls.
The glory, laugh out loud,
was never in the cloud.

On earth, our steady state
will soon depixelate,

our molecules unbinding,
all certainties unwinding,

Till you and I are one,
oh fundamental fun—
divinity from clay,
ta-ra-ra boom-de-ay!

The Acts of Everyone Else

Toby Campion (U.S.)

Apostle-like acts
did not stop
with Paul et al.

Extraordinary
goings-on
happen under

our noses
all the time.
This is not

conjecture.
Yesterday, a
departed lady

saved a boy
by giving him
her heart.

In pandemic
New York,
a doctor kept

hundreds alive
before she died.
In real time,
spirit matters,

our puny
temporality

no match
for the fearless
acts of love

made flesh.
Life eternal
lives inside us.

Waste

Giselle Marks

A waste
of a year,
A waste of our time,
A waste of the sunshine,
A waste of too many lives.
Isolation prevents transmission
But it diminishes all our lives
Yet death is the alternative
If we relax and turn back to normality.
How do we value a life?
How do we value a thousand deaths?
Or ten thousand, a hundred thousand,
When does it become too many?
And when do we start to weep
For people we have never known?
Answers are not flying around
As we try to make sense of a tragedy.
Each death is a waste
Each job lost is a waste
Each human without human contact
Desolate in their misery.

A Demon's Meeting

Dylan Tynan

Isolated to manifest in combining fears,
Though not given the help of listening ears,
No possible resolution for the issues within,
Just repeated isolation full of demons let in,
Hope is stretched, hope is lost, never seeing daylight,
Rather a perpetual metronome of freight.

Sat now in a manifestation of the mind,
Isolation the energy for all demons we come to find,
Converse does the darkness,
Though filling the room with emptiness,
"Seek to destroy not to rebuild,"
"We have them controlled under our hold."

Light is cast upon this room in the soul,
Illuminating it so it cannot be seen now old,
Smiling beams of another's face beam hope,
Loosening the knots with the rope,
Breathing now a world much lighter,
Resolution has come to a fighter.

Are we built to shine?
Is it that we are set to just be fine?
Can help come from ourselves?
Or must we rely of another body of cells?
We are not built a beacon,
We are built as a pillar on which to build.

Pip People

Tom Stockley

in this unprecedented dent
on our collective lives
space is growing for some of us to bloom.
space for we, the chronically anxious
the bent and abandoned
we who never did fit in this world anyway;
and now the world doesn't fit itself.
we, whose idea of a good time
is taking a toaster to a water park
just to see what happens.
we, who have been waiting for a kinder world
since our heart was first broken.
we, who have been tenderised by the meat mallet
    of modern living
the furloughed and forgotten
the ones who thought ourselves rotten to the core
are realising that, all this time,
we were full of pips
tiny cases of infinite potential
sewn in some kind of rubble.
and i know that we'll bloom,
that we'll become orchards
when all of this is over.

Tulips

Nicholas McGaughey

At the trees waving back,
the avenues ghostly with paper blowing
as each day replicates itself.
The birds sing louder with the cars asleep
and the school yard's curfew.

Police patrol two by two,
looking for loiterers
as the sirens blare
and the bells of churches
have no call.

We brood through darkness like tulips
waiting for this blight
to sour another Earth.

Our summer is a winter,
growing infinite crosses
on a steep side of long shadows,
where only small crowds gather.

But in the season after this frost,
I see the spring
shooting upwards to the light,
with petals incandescent
like the bluest star.

The Great Turning

Margot Henderson

This is the time of the great turning
This is the time we've been waiting for
This is the time of the great turning
This is the time for which we were born

This is the time of revolution
This is the time of broken hearts
This is the time of revolution
The time of turning with the stars

This is the time of the great turning
This is the time of coming home
This is the time of the deep soul's yearning
To walk as one and not alone

This is the time of the unraveling
We cannot know how long we have
So let this be the time of gathering
The only thing worth living for is love

This is the time of turning
This is the time of choice
This is the time of learning
To trust our inner voice
This is the time of knowing
We do not walk alone
This is the time of going
Along a path unknown

This is the time of the great turning
A time foretold in prophesy
This is the time of the emerging
The awakened heart of our humanity
This is the time.

Leviathan Stirs

Hadley-James Hoyles

The portraits are placed askew
A gaggle of remembrance requiring
Additional seconds to emerge
From the fug, to integrate the gracious past
With the mildew barricades of the present.

A smile, waterlogged and slouching
Across an entropied face. Silt
Mixing with the cowl of the hermetic ghoul
That is replacing it. Now a frown
Works itself into the architecture of the face.
A tension incorporated to the innate folds
Presented at birth, religned so softly
So subtly, as to dredge up a truth
Never needed until now.

Leviathan stirs, the signs flutter through
The greying trees in springtime.
No helm so bright in the climes, so visceral
As the ageing memorials.
Was it ever so strong, the now? Was it ever
So blinding as the memory reveals?

A gulp from a sacred vessel, to wash away the taste
Of knowing what delves inside
To placate the dwelling of Leviathan. The boards
Maintained in agony, reinforced by bulletins
Streaked across the palatable skies

Of the mind-hive, relenting finally
The mortar's wailing grows weak, and the
Sediment returning to its scarring depths.

No yearning, or chasm rendered hopeful
By the blatant aggression of unyielding life
Of vivacity, can penetrate the aching
Flatness of the newly reworked bones.
A killing song lilts swiftly, across the languid plane
That now becomes the face, the resting
Taken in abandon wrecked and mangled
In the ever intensifying failures of the memory.

What ghosts will dive forth to plug, to bolster up
The gap where Leviathan's stirring can be felt?
Underneath the stretched skin of the smile
That becomes a snarl, what beast
Will presage the great arrival?
And who will know, who of them might care,
Or whom who might care will not know
The lethality that the banal has brought
To this mulching field?

Forgiveness

Muni Subhradip Chakraborty

To learn forgiveness I went to a tree
I asked in whisper what it takes to be
Like a saint who forgives all and more
Like a sea of endless bliss-like purple shore
Or a merry music stream of sublime vast
Nurturing love divine void free of lust.

In whispering murmurs he answered back
Stopping down, he, to his heart, pointed at
Here He is, and He is same everywhere
I see no other , in and around, here or there.
Whom to forgive and forgives then who?
When He alone is there. He hurts, He forgives too.

Solidarity

Tim Turnbull

It's not all Eugene Delacroix, you know,
swanning up the barricades, sporting gun
in hand, chapeau cocked, disordered masses
at your back, swarming toward Elysium.

It's neither a collective swoon in thrall
to the numbing, magniloquent rhetoric
of whichever on-trend demagogue is
presently stowing carpetbag in cart.

It might just, plausibly though, be a hand
on a shoulder, an offer to bear witness
at a board; support in the face of faceless
beadledom, of procedure masking spite;

or only spent shoe-leather; or fortitude
and patience before the gales of windbag
bullies; a gathering up together and
politely, but not mildly, saying no;

grit and the nerve to turn up every week,
or day, notwithstanding weather or disdain;
the will to rally to your friends when asked;
a swig of tea from someone else's flask.

Thin Air

Martin Figura

How can the invisible exist: Gods,
wi-fi, ghosts, society, Ocado, sound?
Are they not all so much hearsay
when they don't cast a shadow?

How can you establish cause and effect
if, when you reach around the back
there are no wires? I've never met
an electrician who wasn't a con artist.

You may as well say it's possible to move
other people's money without ever touching it
and live a very fine life indeed. Sorry,
poor example. Ask me what I see

when I look out of my window and I will tell you
not a single soul. Abstract nouns are only
sentiments. Can I cradle lonely in my arms
and comfort it, for instance? Of course not!

I've read them all Kierkegaard, De Beauvoir,
Schrödinger, Descartes, Sartre, etcetera.
But enlighten me this: if you sealed them
in a room with a brute, who would walk out

on their hind legs at the end of it? Ha!
I thought so. Crack two stones together
until there's a spark. If you're putting faith
in anything at all, I would start there.

Before they wake: a lockdown sunrise

Alison Brackenbury

Red sun hangs perfect, terrible as war,
the blink of grief, the glass which holds no more.
Then gold throbs, the unbearable sun's eye,
magnolia whitens, boiler smoke streams by
till lowered clouds and muffled radiance give
that dull but blessed light by which we live.

Clean

Graham Clifford

We all learn how to make things so clean
they can never be dirty again.

How did we manage before? everyone asks.

Dirt now cannot affix to the shiny surfaces
or any mucky divots.
Even the air gleams.
Anything with a mass is cleaned
at a sub-atomic level.
There are industrial estates
where the dirty is transported in to be cleaned.

In giant hangers they apply the Foam
which does the Job, according to the Procedure
and allowing room for the Ethos.
This whole palaver is considered Man's highest achievement.

Those who can, sense a ripple effect, even in Church.
Even if they don't go.

In time there is discovered a village in the shadow
of a mountain where not everything is clean.
Old books smell of paper being eaten and gum agar.
Bedsheets are seamy.
There is a girl with black, crescents of dirt under her nails
and a knot in her hair from it being dangled in jam.

The sun doesn't get into their valley until late in the morning
and leaves early, so shadow pours in
and they sleep.

Night Thoughts under Lockdown

Paul Isolani Smyth

The night is another country, black and deep
to be awake at night and not to sleep
is like an insect drowning in hot coffee
and therein to swim the dark & foaming creek .

To fall in and to drown
as thoughts flood through my mind ,
to lie awake, awake and yet quite sleepy
is strange and eerie as I lie there bleakly

Night thoughts quite strange can be
the dreams that populate the depths of inner mind
But sleep is the sweet cleanser of the brain
and cleans and clears the thoughts of humankind

To wake up freshly purged of negativity
prepares us to launch forth on fresh activities
and teach ourselves the best way through :
onwards and upwards each fresh day anew .

To positively fight the strains and stresses
that a cruel fate on all of us impresses
To fight and fighting hard to win
O'er all and any ghost or weird goblin.

Emptied

Andrena Zawinski

"...freedom and happiness are found in the flexibility and ease with which we move through change"
Gautama Buddha

The streets and playgrounds, courts and fields are emptied.
The string of row house swings emptied of coffee klatches
across porch rails. Silence on cobbles glistening in morning dew,
heady scent of honeysuckle wafting by windows we peer through.

Framed by the limits of imagination, ears cocked to the sparrow's song,
sun setting on pyramids, creek beds, ice floes, desert flowers,
past our views of the world, ghosts carousing night winds
of our mourning, all the eyes on clear skies boasting stars above

moored cargo ships, snow-capped peaks, the sweaty rainforests.
Our windows view the emptied harbours, farmlands and vineyards,
fire escapes and stoops. All of it emptied of the large and small
of our solitary pleasures in our fractured lives in this godawful air.

Forgive me

David K McDonald

Of all our thoughts we can we say
with words
What makes your soul
Betray the truth, the price to pay

The eyes to see where blind may not
The beat of heart that must not stop

Your reach to touch to feel to hold
That human need forever old

Will our blood course and feed our thoughts
So cold so warm so must
Or God to pray, our right to live
For whose ashes, whose dust

Can we say we gave
the sweetness of giving
we should not save
can we say we passed this way
so cold so cruel so brave
can we say we truly loved and cared
and when our heart will beat no more
can we say forgive me from a lonely grave.

The leftovers

Okorie Harrison

We heard the sound from the north
We got hit from the west
The storm arose from the south
But we finally got victory in the east

The entire world trembled
At the appearance of the mysterious creature
But the foundation of the world stood firm

We were toiled with
And tortured with fear
Tears became a lifestyle
Smiling became what we dream of everyday

It is over
The storm is calmed

We are the leftovers
We will rise again
To see the light of the day
As we sing the songs of victory
And walk in the fullness of liberation.

CHILDREN IN LOCKDOWN

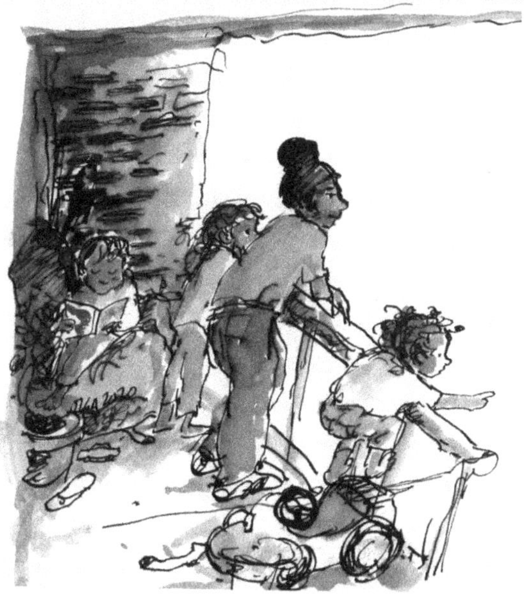

Christine De Luca, Francis H Powell,
Brook Fischer, Olga Solabarrieta

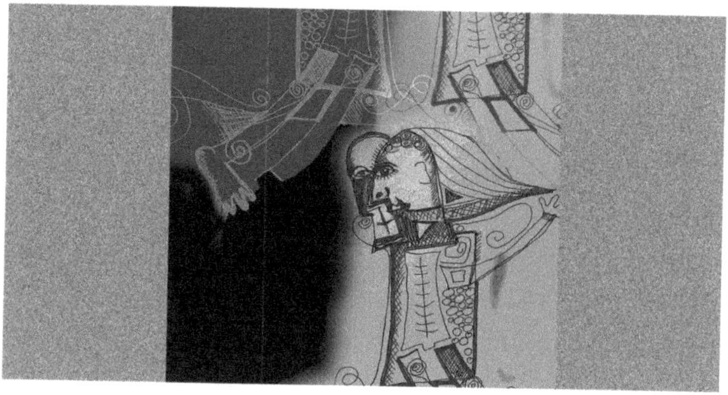

The Daily Ration

Christine De Luca

In the bare carpark a father is teaching his son
to unicycle. The little boy is all a flap, trying
his balance on the air. Soon he is winging it,
engrossed and delighted; pedalling, then
catching the ball, throwing it back.
The father can speed up, slow down, backpedal,
scoop up the ball like a polo player. Tomorrow,
the child will do likewise. Meanwhile
his sister is perfecting her keepie-uppies,
counting into herself, enthralled; happy
to tolerate a younger brother, unphased
by a father in shorts, without his usual tie.
They teeter but do not fall: time to pedal
forwards, wordless, back into the world.

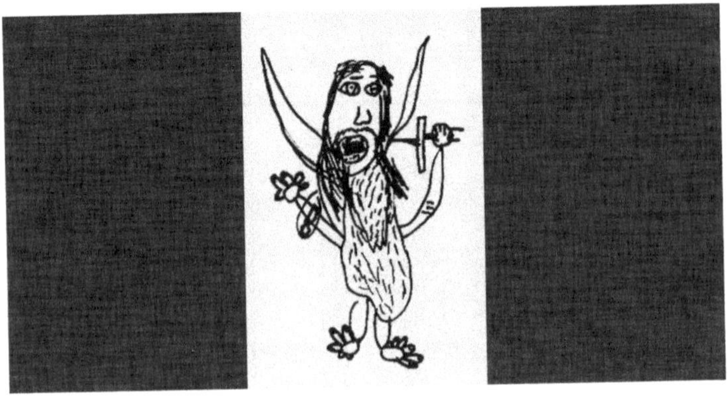

Innocence

Francis H Powell

Oh little beating heart of innocence
with your gentle tugs of curiosity
The value of which, knows no bounds
For you this damned bug
can be eliminated with a well-aimed ray gun
and God is up there fighting for us with his sword and shield
You said to me today the clouds look like monsters
well we all need to be warriors
from time to time
Every day is a new opening
and please excuse me when I lose my temper
for not everything is your fault
being huddled together in our house
There's you and me and your mother
then there's the dog, all trying to make sense
of what is happening as well as satisfying different needs
Nobody can fault your endeavour

You might trip and fall
but you can always get up
and don't be put off by the cynics
who trawl through the ashes of doom
If you plant many seeds
one will surely grow into an arboreal wonder.

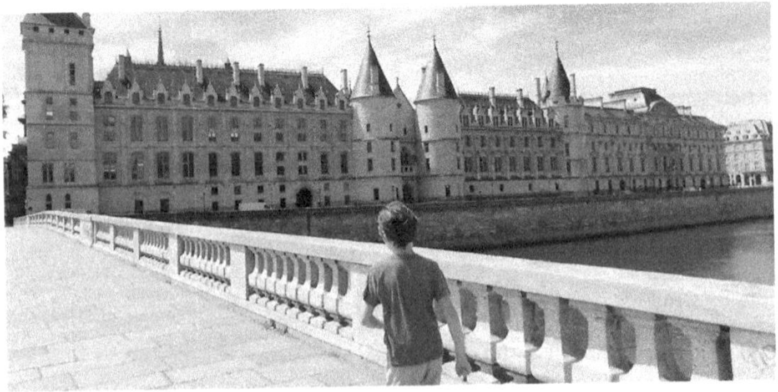

Traverse

Brook Fischer

A boy named after a river
Crosses a river, deep in thought
Barely registering the barren bridge
Or his adoring brother and anxious mother padding just a few paces behind him
The eerie emptiness of Paris and the fear of airborne pathogens are silently acknowledged by one, then suppressed
Day after day, they traverse the Marais
(And occasionally the Seine)
Relishing one hour of freedom
One kilometer of discovery
Today they notice tiny, pale pink blossoms peeking out from behind a wrought iron fence near Notre Dame
Oh the healing nuances of nature
The phone emits soft, tinkling notes
A signal to return home
Home is a small but safe space
For two energetic boys, equipped with their toys
And just enough naïveté to shield the mind during a pandemic.

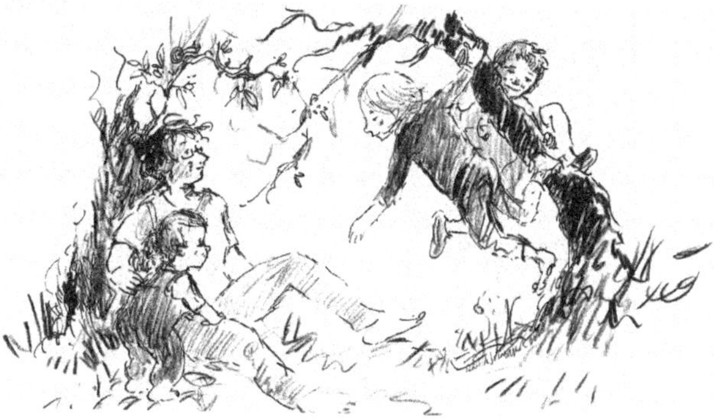

My Three Moonbeams

Olga Solabarrieta

The world has gone mad
Masks and steriliser
And now plastics back
But you
You three shining gems
You dig in the ground and play;
You scrape, you mix and then play some more

The world has gone mad
Counting the dead
And waiting for more
But you
You sparkling raindrops
You sing you chatter and play;
You cry, you mimic and then play some more

The world has gone mad
We have to stay home
Or else fill in a form

But you
You three bright firecrackers
You make clay food, rabbit houses and play;
gather up kindling, burn a fire and then play some more

The world has gone mad
And you don't mind
Three sweet moonbeams that shine
All day and glow in the night.

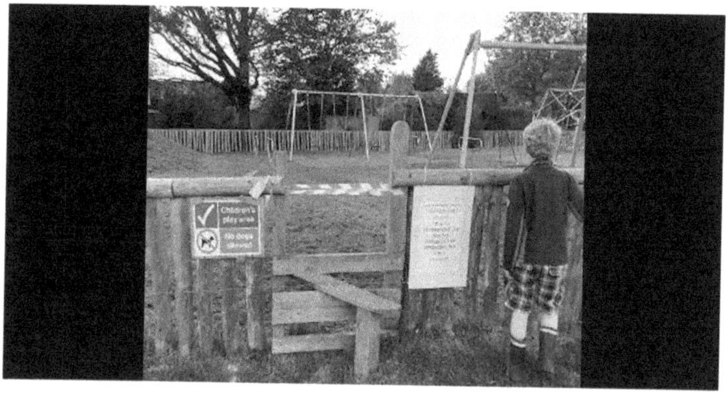

Cordoned Off

Francis H Powell

An Empty space
where cries of happiness
would normally call out
where parents normally
watch their brood
as they run about
with a whir of energy
A boy looks on
trying to rationalize it all
surveying what is his normal domain
Oh William what are you thinking?
in that deep thoughtful head of your yours
As swings lay static
locked and motionless
perhaps a bird calls out
or there is the occasional murmur of traffic
Even the sky shouts out "emptiness"
all lies dormant.

Ode to Son

Francis H Powell

I have to keep you from harm's way
well away from the lurking danger
but I know you need to run and move
and let off your boundless energy
that bottles up inside you
like a dormant volcano

You are confined and restricted
perhaps confused by what is happening
You are limited to a walk with the dog
who at least gives you pleasure and joy
but chains have been put in place
that hold back the wings
that let you fly.

LOVE IN LOCKDOWN

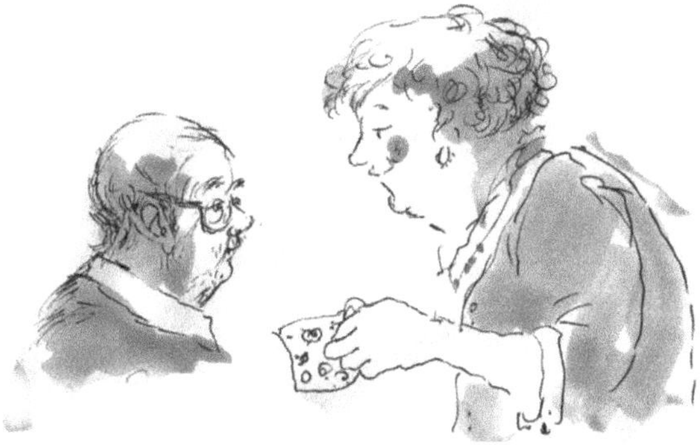

Leela Soma, Francis H Powell,
Suki Spangles, Neil Zetter,
Bernard Young

Claps

Leela Soma

Thirty-five claps to Christmas
How we count our days now?
Surreal to imagine the fairy lights
On dark November nights, shops
Ablaze, people fighting over new toys.

Days stretch as we look out the window
Watch an empty sun-streaked street
Itch to go out and drive to the coast
Feel the sea breeze on our skin, dig our
Toes in the hot sand as we lick a 99 cone

Images that seem out of reach, yet this
Maybe a transient phase, a golden time
To be with our loved ones, spend hours
Baking, playing Monopoly, listening to
Each other understanding that our basic
Need is love, kindness and more love.

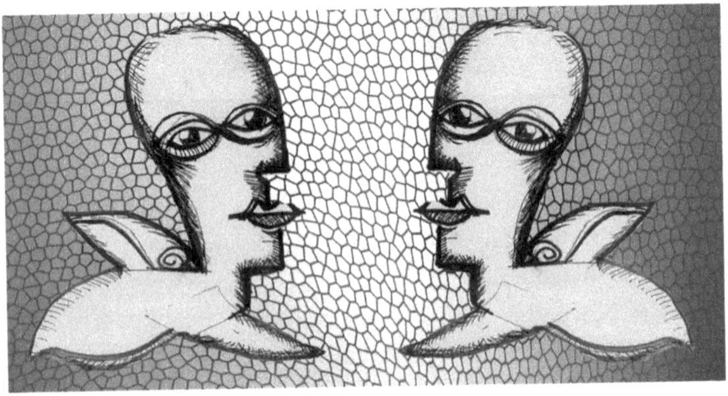

Dating Covid 19-Style

Stephanie Davidson

They said …
You're not allowed to go out during lockdown
Not even the single and free
So I dove down to fish for a loophole
And emerged victoriously
You see …
The loophole was right there before me
In the clippings and cuttings and ash
So this morning I took out the weeds
And tonight I'm gonna take out the trash.

Love in the time of Corona

Suki Spangles

around nine-thirty in the evening
the setting sun peach melba
masked like a bank robber skiing
i had to be somewhere
a nowhere to be precise
the police did not stop me
wearing a mask it is presumed is only basic good manners now
it means you are a taxpayer
a moving piece of herd-wallpaper
or it means you are a very cunning bank robber
pretending to be a taxpayer blending in endorsing
    the absurdist theatre
and so i journeyed thus to a faceless building
tilting at facial recognition cameras
the night was young and she was waiting
with a pump-action sanitizer
just like in the movies
or maybe not..

in the distance a couple holding hands
were ambling in my direction
lovers strolling in the eerie emptied streets
they saw me and...*a beat...*
elegantly danced a few metres apart from one another
slow-step and a quarter turn each way
an invisible daisy chain stretched between them
about two metres

so that one end pulled near me
and by their air-bubble rosary i was glanced a ming vase ricochet..
and after passing them
i turned to see their concertina contract
then part. then contract
confounding another passing stranger
with or without a mask...

The Garden Wall

Francis H Powell

The garden wall loomed tall and bushes were full with leaves. Her garden was rugged, some might say it needed attention. However it brought her joy, it was her possession, nobody else's. At the far end of the garden was a cherry tree, which for a short period was covered in white frothy blossom. It was to her mind the jewel of the garden, despite the fact it did not provide her with many cherries, which for the most part were devoured by greedy birds. There was a rope hanging from one branch, and in summer she could laze in an hammock chair, sheltered from the sun, either reading or just passing the time away.

Surrounding the tree was long grass and some wildflowers, including columbines, harebells, cornflowers, fox-gloves, and, depending on the time of year, wild daffodils. The lawn was shaggy and unkempt, with moss creeping and spreading like an uncontrolled fire. There was an inundation of ivy. She brought some decorations for the garden, ceramic pots and urns, as well as small ethnic sculptures - nothing of any value, but to her they added some character. Both sides of the lawn were lined with an incongruous assortment of flowers and a spindly rose bush that produced orange flame roses. She had a wooden wine barrel full of kale, swiss chard and mustard greens. She brought some rustic garden furniture and would eat outside when the weather permitted.

She'd bought the house to live with her partner at the time, but as they were about to move in together he'd walked out on her. She had wondered, from time to time when they were together, if he was really the type who would manage the toils of a committed relationship. Of course he was great fun, amusing, pleasant to be with, but not the type to have to deal with the practical side of life, the humdrum things everybody has to do, part of the daily grind.

Once their relationship got too serious, it was time for him move on; he'd got cold feet, the fun of the relationship died down when too many elements of practicality crept in. He had left her a handwritten note. In truth, it hadn't amounted to much. At first the overall feeling was sadness, but then anger had set in. Once she read it a few times to take the words in, she screwed it up in her hand and hurled it at her bin in disgust. Then she sat down and wept.

The letter contained about four sentences, it must have taken him a few minutes to scrawl. Lana, I am just writing to say, I am not sure I can carry on our relationship. I have been thinking things over, and I am not sure we are right for each other. I know this is not great timing, but I am afraid I have little choice but to end the relationship, before we really commit and make a terrible mistake.

Thankfully, she had enough money to get by; it was more the fact that the house they were supposed to share would be empty with his absence. She'd had to tell all her friends and family, of course they had all been sympathetic, but this was barely any form of genuine compensation. Getting over this bombshell hadn't been easy, days of waking up alone, staring at the ceiling, feeling empty inside.

They had visited the house together, he'd been most enthusiastic, repeating over and over "it's perfect Lana", imagining how it could be modernized. It had belonged to an old woman; she had lived there most of her life and it showed with the decoration. It was like a canvas; a painter needed to infuse new life into the dated décor. In truth it was drab, somewhat comatose, as if it had been dormant for years and needed invigorating.

Lana, once settled in, set about making modifications, trying to make it more her house, to whittle away the remnants of the previous owner. The old woman died and her son wanted to sell the property. He lived far away and was just happy to pocket the money and have the property off his hands. There had been some bargaining before he finally had accepted Lana's offer. Lana had bought a bottle of champagne which she shared with her soon to be ex-partner, Max.

She should have paid more attention to Max's reputation of walking out of relationships; he'd been married once and had a young son Ollie, who he saw every other weekend. Lana had even grown fond of Ollie, and he had obviously warmed to her, so this had added to her bitter disappointment. She tried her best to obliterate Max from her mind, but it wasn't easy, his absence left a big hole.

She didn't know any of the neighbours and her house was at the end of the road, leaving only one immediate neighbour. Between her and this neighbour was an imposing wall and a lot of foliage. After she had moved in, it was apparent this neighbour was absent from their property, only visiting some weekends. Was this neighbour a man or a woman? Were they young or old, there was no way of telling. When there was any sign of this neighbour, she heard the lawn being cut or some sign they were pruning some plant or pottering about in their garden. She never heard this person's voice, they didn't seem to invite visitors and lived like her - alone. All that foliage meant she couldn't put a face to them. She imagined perhaps they would leave their houses at the same moment or perhaps return, meaning they would finally meet, but this didn't seem to happen.

On weekends Lana liked to get away from her new house, staying with her family or friends, anything to break her now lonely existence. She had always been used to company, she had three sisters and a brother. She was the youngest and her siblings had always doted on her. She had lots of nephews and nieces who she loved to see, and she longed to start a family of her own, but Max had dashed that hope. Maybe this was another reason he left her, he suspected that living together might mean she would get broody, she had talked about what their children would look like. Max quickly shut the conversation down, changing the subject, his face told her many things. It was clear he drew the line at having any more children. He had enough responsibilities with one child and having to pay maintenance to his ex-wife after a grimy divorce.

Having mourned Max's loss after a painful healing process, Lana began to levitate towards the idea that she should seek a new partner. Friends had tried to encourage her and had even introduced her to some of their single male friends, unfortunately none really had captured Lana's interest. Was she too choosy? She had tried, in desperation, online dating and had gone on a few dates. The men often looked nothing like their pictures, some were considerably older, or their pictures glorified their prosaic looks, and their profiles didn't allude to some most annoying habits.

James Pembleton (was that his real name she wondered) claimed he was a stockbroker earning lots of money, in fact money was the mainstay of his conversation. She saw him rev off in a car that looked like it was set for the scrap heap, and some of his stories just didn't add up. He had given her a business card and she'd researched the company he allegedly worked for, it had ceased trading three years ago. What a fraud, what a creep.

Tony Bandanna, hair obviously dyed, took it for granted she would want to bed him on their first date. Nothing could have been further from the truth. Tony was an on-off actor, but more off than on, it was clear. He had been to drama school, one Lana had never heard of, and had been on television, a few bit parts - blink and you would miss him. He was a nobody who thought he was a somebody. He talked all the time about his mother, it was obvious he still had a strong bond with her, that she was still the dominant feature in his life.

They had eaten dinner in an Indian restaurant, the food had been pleasant, but Lana was only too happy to slip away from Tony. He had arrived with a big bunch of roses. He was tanned, wearing a colourful patterned shirt, and Lana quickly suspected she had been duped by his photograph and profile. Another fake, another loser. He often laughed after every remark he made, snorting at the end of the sentence.

At first she had forced herself to smile, but soon found herself cringing. Tony began to quote Shakespeare, "She's beautiful, and therefore to be wooed; She is woman, and therefore to be won." Well Lana was not to be won, she paid her part of the bill. She said she had to get up early for work the next day and, despite his persistence, managed to get home. She told her friend Sally about her date with Tony, who had made her skin crawl, the pair of them laughed about it, in retrospect it had been funny. In truth some of her dates could have been married, with four children, looking for more excitement in their dull suburban lives, Lana could never sort the truth from the lies.

One man, Simon, had interested her, unlike all the others. He didn't talk that much or set out to impress her. He seemed awkward, like he was finding dating strangely taxing. They met in a wine bar. There had been some long silences, Lana had tried to work out how to break this wall of silence. Simon was intense, like there was a big weight always on his mind. He told her he read a lot of books and did a bit of gardening. He had once been engaged to be married, but he and his fiancé never went through with it, delaying it, mulling over it, and consequently over time they had drifted apart. He'd regretted this, his indecision killed their relationship. Simon taught literature in a university. Lana was surprised he was single, but then again, he was incredibly shy and deep thinking, and this might ward off a lot of women. He wasn't overly good looking, and had a scar on his left cheek, but at the same time he was somehow attractive to Lana. He was so understated compared to any of the other men she had met. There was something about him she felt bound to discover.

He had taken her telephone number and email address, but all she had received was a curt email, with no indication that he wanted to see her, or that there was anything good that had come out of their evening together. His response left her disappointed. She returned his email with an equally brusque response.

She gave up on him, she was afraid to invest emotionally in him, worried he wouldn't give anything to her in exchange. He was a confused soul, a man lost in a sea of ambivalence. Life went on but she never seemed to meet anybody who equalled Simon.

The confinement had come into force. Lana was now even more isolated, hours by herself. There was her job to keep her occupied but sitting in front of a computer without human contact soon began to grind her down. Time moved slowly. Days became repetitive, the same routines. The news every day was more distressing. Life had taken a new turn and it wasn't a nice one. At least she had her garden, and when the weather was pleasant she could go out and potter about. Sometimes she was aware of her "neighbour". He or she was also ensconced. Still no signs of who this person might be. She was tempted to call out, "Hello, I am your neighbour, my name is Lana, who are you?" This idea seemed ridiculous and she would be embarrassed, never live it down. Instead there remained this wall of non-communication

One day there was talk on the news of an impending storm. The wind indeed had picked up and rain fell in biblical-like proportions. Her garden was battered. The storm seemed to stay for a couple of days, playing havoc. There were leaves and broken parts of bushes strewn all over her lawn. She cleared them up. One morning while she was sat by her computer, she heard the constant drone of a machine. Her neighbour was cutting away at some of the bushes. She felt compelled to investigate.

There was an indistinct face of a man. Before long she would be able to fully make out his face. He was cutting away at damaged branches, anyway in truth the bush needed pruning. She stood mesmerised. Finally, his identity was about to be revealed.

A branch fell into her garden. "Oh sorry" a voice called out. It was a voice she recognized. Her heart pounded. Her mind was in a flux of disbelief. It was of all people... Simon.

"Oh, hello Lana," he said in a dry voice, as if nothing surprising had occurred, that it was no coincidence they were living next to one another, as if everything was normal.

"Wow Simon!" Lana had exclaimed showing far more emotion.

"Just clearing away some branches damaged by the storm," he said in his equally dead pan manner, taking a break from his work.

"Have you lived here long," Lana demanded.

"Not exactly," he replied, "in fact this house was where my mother lived, but she is in hospital, so with this lockdown, I thought I should live here and look after it. She has rather let it go to rack and ruin and it needs some attention."

"Oh, I see," Lana said.

"I like your garden Lana," Simon said, peering about.

"I am no real gardener," Lana said modestly.

"Have you lived here long?" Simon asked.

"Not that long, I bought it a couple of years back, I am still doing work on it."

"Yeah houses do take up a lot time," Simon sighed; wiping some sweat off his forehead.

"I suppose I had better let you get on," Lana said, imagining he might be impatient to get on with the work he'd been doing, until she had interrupted him.

"I don't know, it's great to talk to another person, apart from on the telephone. It is very limiting, this confinement." Lana was shocked, she never expected him to wish to speak more to her. They had chatted for half an hour or more, until a few drops of rain had begun to fall and they both ventured inside.

Lana was kind of stunned by what had occurred and she was hardly able to remain focussed on her work. It led her to venture out into the garden on a more regular basis, in the hope that she might be able to engage in another conversation. The cloud of loneliness was somewhat lifted, knowing that Simon was not far away, only separated from her by a wall. The rest of the day, he seemed to be cocooned in his house, never venturing out. The next morning a similar pattern followed, it was both disappointing and frustrating to Lana.

In the afternoon she was sat at her computer, when suddenly she heard her name being called. She was surprised, she rose out of her seat and went into the garden, only to see Simon on the other side smiling.

"Hey Lana, how are you doing? I fancied a chat, if you're not too busy?"

"Not bad" Lana stuttered, wincing at a sudden burst of sunlight.

"I would invite you in for a coffee, but it's not allowed." Simon said, laughing at his own remark.

"I guess not," answered Lana, adding, "I could invite you over for a glass of chilled wine and some canapés, if you are in the mood, but I won't. The neighbours might talk."

"We can't have that," Simon said, adding, "so we will just have to get used to chatting over this garden wall."

"I suppose you are right, perhaps I should get a garden chair, it might be more comfortable, and you could get a chair," Lana suggested. It seemed a bit absurd. the two sat down, facing one another, with distance and that wall a barrier between them.

As time passed by their relationship grew stronger. Lana would call Simon for a rendezvous in the garden and vice versa. She prepared meals for him, he would send over a basket on a rope and she would fill it with food. He would suggest books for her to read, written by authors she had never heard of, and when she had read them, they would discuss them, both offering their opinions.

During one encounter over the garden wall, he had referred back to their date.

"I was foolish, as usual, I should have followed things up. As usual I prevaricated. The thing was, you reminded me of somebody special and this perturbed me."

"Oh really" Lana replied, intrigued.

"Yes, you resemble Rose. I was engaged to her, but we never got married."

"I think you mentioned this," Lana said, "but you never mentioned that I reminded you of her." This revelation slightly worried Lana; would she be a secondary replacement for his previous love? On the other hand, he obviously recognized something in her that he was clearly drawn to, there was a link. Also, in a way, everybody gets haunted by their previous, meaningful relationships, which cling to their minds.

If only these were normal times, Lana thought, they could be together, but the truth was they were separated by a garden wall and forbidden from getting close to one another. Time would tell if there was something developing between them. When the restrictions were lifted, the relationship would truly be put to the test. Somehow, Lana thought there was something special about Simon. They had connected with their minds.

Love in a Covid Climate

Neal Zetter

What rule did I transgress
What crime did I commit
For you to smash my heart
Into the smallest bits?
It's splintered, shattered on the floor
You cut me to my very core
Remotely you walked out the door
Now you don't Zoom me anymore

We used to chat for hours
(Once I'd clicked on your link)
In our respective beds
Curled up with just a drink
With online love you knew the score
I want things as they were before
But I'm a shipwreck far from shore
Now you don't Zoom me anymore

Was my wifi too weak?
My video unclear?
My background indistinct?
My voice too quiet to hear?
Did I break some unwritten law?
All of my invites are ignored
What happened to our great rapport?
Now you don't Zoom me anymore

I thought you were the one
Since our first virtual date
Till 'old normal' resumed
The physical could wait
Our romance clearly had a flaw
I punch my keypad, fingers raw
You've changed your number – final straw!
Now you don't Zoom me anymore

(And although I remain your true believer
You don't FaceTime, WhatsApp, Skype or Instagram me
Either).

Love In The Time Of Lockdown

Bernard Young

Meals: cooked. Clothes: washed. Plans:
squashed. But shirts dry in the sun.
Yes, the sun shines, even at a time like this.
And the two of us continue to laugh, hug, kiss

and get a little irritable. Something new:
my back aches now. It never used to!
We phone. Write emails. Send texts
and worry about what might happen next.

We catch up on TV (Killing Eve, Mum, The Crown)
and find old films to watch again (Moonrise Kingdom,
The Sting , The Dressmaker, Lost In Translation
starring Bill Murray and Scarlett Johansonn).

We read. Me: 'Emergency Kit: Poems for Strange
Times' edited by Jo Shapcott and Matthew Sweeney.
She: 'Educated' by Tara Westover.
There's a picture of a young girl on a swing on its cover.

We check the online news. We slip out
when no one else is about.
We hold gloved hands when we walk.
We breathe in deeply. And talk. And talk.

HOPE AND DESPAIR

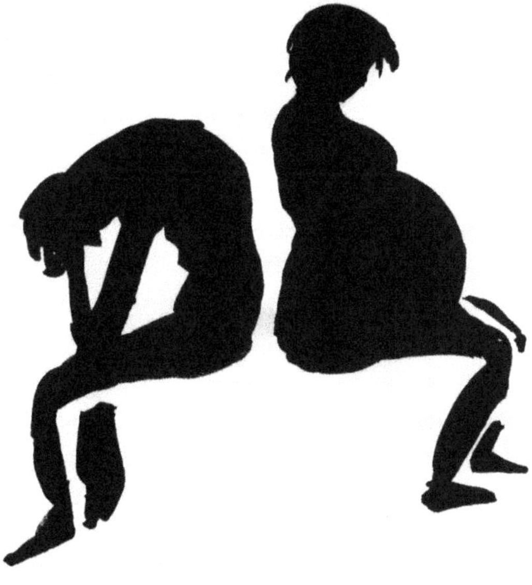

Lynda Scott Araya, Chris White, Josiane Vincent, Hélène Argo, Tiffany Apan, Francis H Powell, Leela Soma, Sophie Jane Winter, Shannon Pratuch, Linda Watkins, Christopher T Dabrowski, Thomas Stockley, Margot Henderson, Adele C. Geraghty

Fraught

Lynda Scott Araya

"Where am I?"
I wake,
cocooned in blankets
Marooned in darkness.
Unsure of my direction
My bearings in a world
Unknown.
Upside down.
"You're here"
Says my husband.
He touches my head gently
Turns me to face the bedroom door
Under which the insidious
pandemic
Creeps.

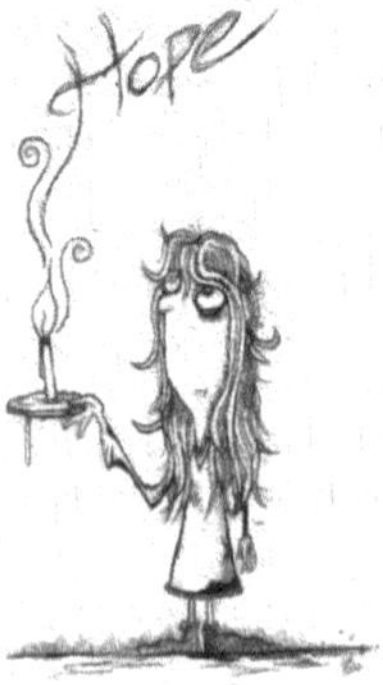

Hope

Chris White

It's the smile that you swap with a stranger
That wave from across the street
The stretching and yawning, first thing in the morning
Then hitting that floor with your feet
It's the ghost that we all cling on to
When we feel like we just cannot cope
The candle at night, the dark tunnel's light
That warm arm around you is
Hope.

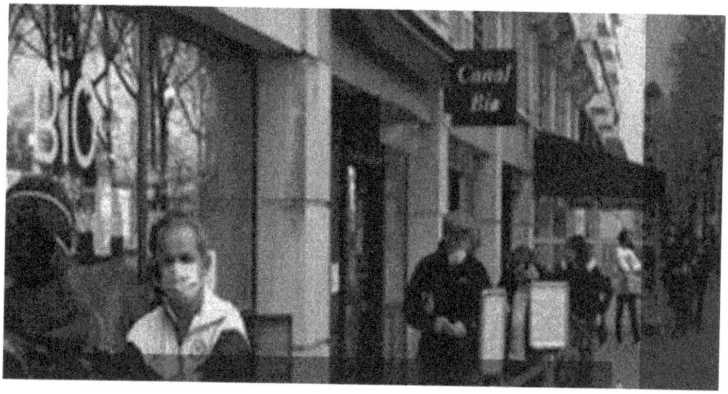

In the line

Josiane Vincent

Black and white
To tell the plight of humanity
Under the spell of mischievous hands
Sowing sorrow
The phantasmagorical scene of
A gagged figure's endless procession
Motionless
Within a narrow corridor
Enclosed
between barriers and walls
Reveals a tale of desolation
The carnival
A forlorn memory
Has lost its permissive lustre
This sorrowful line of estranged beings
With restrictions/instructions
As sole horizon
Draws a pitiful picture
Tell me it's just a bad dream
Tell me it's a mirage
That will soon vanish.

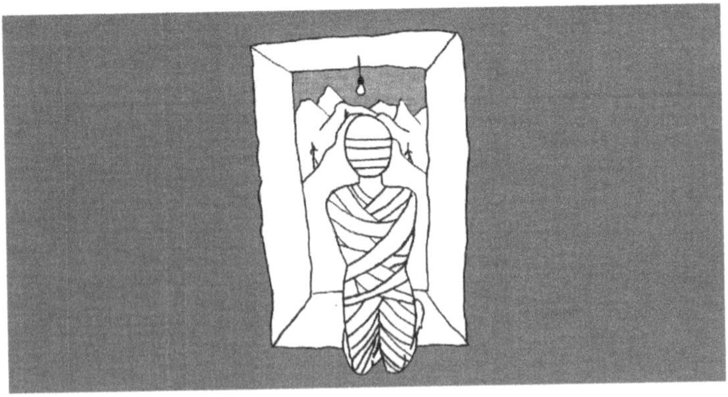

Queen in Babylon

Hélène Argo

Four walls shelter me from the rain,
All slaps of the wind of life,
from the rays of the sun I'm shielded
as well as from both man and beast
but sometimes I miss their company
Four walls where on certain days
the dusty remnants of the outside world
Come attached underfoot
From those who still love me and still visit me.

At dusk, I'm in Babylon
A noble queen with a mournful look:
It's the promised life for me if I stay good.
Hatching in my sanctuary, I have exceeded your limits
And sadness has slipped away
Only two separate lives for the same person.
Two separate lives in Babylon.

Four walls that sometimes turn
At times quickly all around me;
Those in white coats lose their heads then stand still
Frozen clean by a double dose.
Four soft walls like a sheep's wool
Whose thick fleece sponges my rage,
Whose passive resistance is the worst of cages,
Sometimes, as if possessed, I laugh.

But at dusk, I'm in Babylon
A noble queen with a sorrowful look:
It's the promised life if I stay good.
Hatching in my straightjacket, I have exceeded your limits
And nothing remains of my sad state,
Only two separate lives for the same person.
Two separate lives in Babylon.

Four ramparts still under attack
By mad fevers, my enemy sisters.
I lie down, they remain lurking;
I'm waiting for a dream to guide me to Babylon.

Rebirth

Tiffany Apan

In the darkness there is light
From the ashes the phoenix will rise
We will rebirth
We will be reborn
Dig through a ditch of rocks
For the treasure on the other side
Setting out on the quest
Continuing through this dark night
We will rebirth
We will be reborn
Through the storm clouds
The sun will come out
Warming Terra with golden rays
After the rain washes away all pain
We will rebirth
We will be reborn
Setting on a quest, continuing through the night
In the dark there is always light
And from the ashes a phoenix will rise.

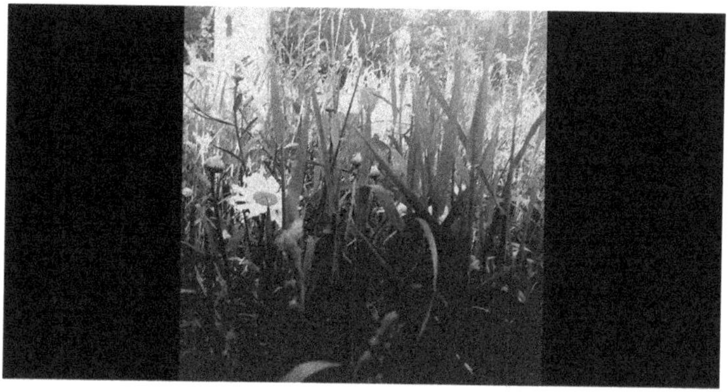

Rhapsody in summer

Francis H Powell

A rhapsody in summer
The announcement of a new born child
with a perfect future mapped out.
A long wistful meander
As drops of silvery rain,
race from yielding skies
anointing our heads
nurturing our happiness
The constellations of stars
at the wake of the night
The planets in perfect formation
Silvery shadows,
gilded by moonlight
A band of troubadours
playing a masterful tune
as gypsies dance round

a fire, with flames the colour
of azurian blue.
Hands touch flesh
as soft as dolphin's fins
bodies quiver in delirious pleasure
I walk through the eye of a storm
I walk on burning coals
through a pit of vipers
a vat of oil, simmering heat
a garland of sharpened knives
no evil do I fear
not one injury to report
All is unblemished
Days span out
like wondrous dreams
Fires burn, throughout the night
Tenderness is shown across the minions
All are drawn in a whirl of creativity
Fused by the lights of the stars.
Old hearts grow new
in a flurry of regeneration
as breaking waves
gently rumble, close to the shore
Good news is passed on by Mercury himself
While bathing in an ocean of crystalline lather.
Conversations are laced with splatters of good will
humor and empathy and witty refrain
All of this as we wander, our way home
Such bliss and pleasure in our hands to keep.
The spiral, the vortex,
the Tibetan bell
all sing like a celestial choir

as trinkets drop gently from the skies
landing in the hands of the needy
no need to rummage for food
as all is of plenty
Oh if this day could come today
We could all walk so tall and proud
and share in the life of the gods.

Sorrow

Leela Soma

Sorrow has elegance,
a colourless canvas,
shades of aquarelle,
pale in their grief
denial, anger,
'why me?' heart asks
as it searches for the
familiar in clothes,
a faint smell on the pillow
seeking solace in prayers,
bereft, tears
flow unknowingly,
the void remains,
the blue of the corona'd lungs,
veined as a scar,
buried in the recesses
of the soul
unspeaking,
volumes muted
alphabets unstrung,
words become superfluous,
loss tied to words,
a language with which
we learn to laugh, talk,
cry and mourn,
orphaned words
hushed, a quiet
numb, heart aches
the hurt waiting
for time to heal.

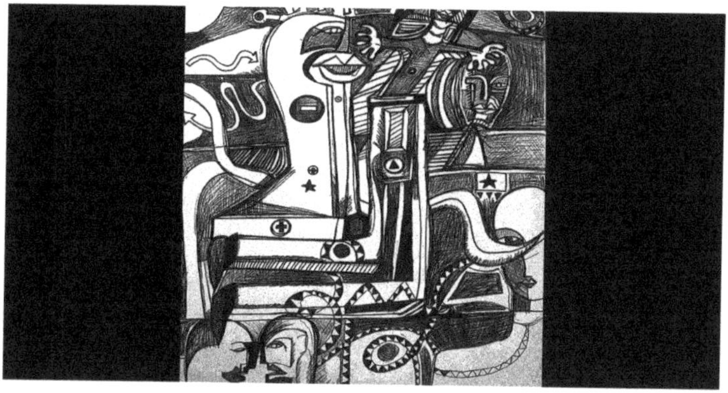

You are not alone

Sophie Jane Winter

Shut the church doors
Put on your gloves
Close the cafes
The clock strikes 5
They bellow: YOU ARE NOT ALONE

Don't cough
How rude!
Tick, tick, tick, tock
No time for bullshit
Stop your commute,
You silly fool
Don't visit your grandad!
Stay away, stay away!
Laugh at the panic buyers
Panic buy.
Halt the service sector
It's not that important anyway...

The clock strikes 5
They bellow: YOU ARE NOT ALONE

Is your journey essential?
Are you essential?
We won't be like Italy
Tick tock
We are not America
Block the schools
Stop the cleaners
Our beast
Our greed,
Did you know it can be paused!
Silence
A COVID Community
We've lost our jobs.
No footsteps
No planes
Is this a message
Is it a dream?
The clock strikes 5
They bellow: YOU ARE NOT ALONE

Righty-tighty
Stiffen your lip
Log onto zoom let's do a quiz
You can still buy fizz!
Still shop in a Marks and Sparks!
People are kinder
And there's less...
Less noise
Less stress.
A message pops up

Apologies
We're decreasing your interest
The clock strikes 5
They bellow: YOU ARE NOT ALONE

Skeleton workers
Stop going to the parks
You irresponsible parent of 3!
One in one out!
Our lovely British police
They can stop you now.
While munching through your tins,
Keep clapping for the NHS
Beans, tuna, tomatoes
Any spare?
Tick, tick, tick, tock
The prime ministers got it
The clock strikes 5
They bellow: YOU ARE NOT ALONE

He looks tired,
manages to crack a joke
It's still a novelty
It's corporate socialism
'Don't let your staff go'
'We'll pay them'.
Tick tock
April showers have arrived
We get to be contemplative now,
behind the pages of a book.
We forgot to mention,
Not now
(for goodness sake)

'We didn't say we could pay them now!'
Redundancy.
I can hear the birds
I can feel the trees, breathing
Some people's homes
Are in their head.
Some homes are prisons
Poorly designed,
for isolation.
The clock strikes 5
They bellow: YOU ARE NOT ALONE.

The Hoarders

Francis H Powell

Harry Hoarder, woke up with a start. His wife Aida, who lay next to him in their king-size bed, was still gently snoring, a repetitive nasal rumbly sound, accompanied by an occasional snort. Aida went to sleep wearing a hairnet, lest she shed some of her locks during the night. She loved her house and wanted it to be spick and span. The mound that was Aida, did not stir as Harry hurriedly got out of bed, took a quick shower, then went downstairs to the kitchen. He put, as always, one and a half spoons of coffee into his mug and switched on the kettle. He turned on the television to capture news updates. There wasn't any talk of food shortages, but with the kind of situation that was developing, Harry reckoned they were on the way and he wanted to be ahead of the game.

He was a man who was always making calculations. He calculated how long ten toilet rolls would last - fifty-three days, unless he or Aida succumbed to some stomach virus. Toilet paper, he thought, was a must. If forced to use paper towels, the toilet could block up and a plumber would have to be called.

The Hoarders didn't have children, which in a way was a blessing in this present crisis, as children to Harry's mind were unpredictable creatures, who might add an extra expense, here and there and the frugal Hoarders weren't the types to splash out on any add-ons caused by any Hoarder offspring. Harry had read in a respectable newspaper, what with the cost of childcare and education costs, the average investment in raising a child to the age of 21 in Britain would be approximately £231,843 and to Harry's mind, this would be money not well spent.

Harry's brother Bill had children (perhaps many). There were four official Hoarders and despite being grown-up and some with jobs, they still scrounged off their father, Harry and Aida, had been round Bill's house and seen this with their own eyes. Everything the Hoarders bought was carefully written down in a book. Harry could tell you the last time he had bought a can of Coke and how much it had cost. The Hoarders often had arguments, Harry accusing Aida of unnecessary spending, or vice versa, but generally the Hoarder's house was well run and even in this crisis, it would continue to be so. The Hoarders knew how to live with limits imposed. They remembered the post war years when they had been young children

Harry recalled that food rationing in Britain had ended at midnight on 4 July 1954, and the Hoarder household had celebrated, his father tossing a ration book on the fire, in a rare act of insubordination. His father was a butcher and the price of meat had soared, but the Hoarders had eaten rashers of bacon and real eggs. The war mentality of scrimping and saving had been imprinted on both Harry and Aida's minds as well as saving up for a "rainy day." It seemed a prolonged rainy day was on the horizon. When they married some thirty years ago, Aida had made her wedding dress out of some old curtains that were a bit frayed at the bottom.

She had, in Harry's mind, looked wonderful, but had invited quite a few comments like "haven't I seen that material before?" by people who were aware of her parent's house décor. Her aunt Sally was a baker and had made the cake and of course Harry's father had provided the meat. Bill was the best man but had disgraced himself, getting very drunk and was later found in an uncompromising situation with one of the young bridesmaids, who he had managed to seduce with his mannish charms. Harry and Aida hadn't ventured abroad for their honeymoon, as Harry was still in the army. Instead, the couple had stayed two nights together in a hotel in Blackpool, walking along the sea front, hand in hand, buying the occasional ice cream, before Harry went back to his duties and Aida set up home in the army barracks. It was a rather bleak house, but Aida had tried to jolly it up, but with limited effect.

When Harry was in the army, Aida did not adapt well to being a soldier's wife and had missed her family - her parents and five sisters. When discharged, Harry became a salesman, selling vacuum cleaners, door-to-door. With a beaming smile, he convinced bored housewives that their lives would be changed if they purchased the fantastic product he was offering. But now, Harry was retired and, in truth, often bored.

He had his dog, Rufus, to walk every day. And on Thursday's, he went to the ex-servicemen club where he would moan about the price of food and the reprobate youth of today. He watched racing on television and, when Aida was being negligent or away visiting one of her sisters, he might put on a bet. He'd never won much, but it added something to his humdrum life, that he might one day, if the gods looked down on him and one of his bets came good.

Occasionally he would go and see Bill, whose life had proved chaotic. Bill had been married three times and had quite a few affairs besides. He, in truth, took after Harry's father, who had won over more than a few women's hearts, with promises of extra rations. His mother was aware of his father's wandering eyes and unscrupulous ways but had soldiered on with their marriage in a most servile and honourable manner.

Harry had a third brother, Jason, who he had lost contact with. Jason had married a middle-class woman called Jasmine. Jason was great tennis player and had met his wife at the local tennis club. They had become tennis partners, and had struck up an unlikely relationship. Afterwards, Harry noticed a change come over Jason. He no longer joined his brothers down at the pub for a sing-along and some laughs. He began talking of plays that he'd seen and books with strange long titles by authors that Harry had never heard of. Before long Jason secured a place at the local university, having passed some exams and studied at home, absorbing book after book. Harry and Bill had been invited to Jason and Jasmine's wedding, mostly out of obligation. It had been a lavish affair, but both Harry and Bill had felt unwelcome and mostly ignored. Harry had noted how Jasmine's friends had turned their noses up at him and Aida. Some had even laughed at Aida's dress, hardly bothering to disguise their mirth.

At first the brothers had exchanged Christmas cards with brief messages, but soon even this tenuous ritual began to disappear. Now Jason could be living on the other side of the world and Harry wouldn't even know it. He wondered if he would recognize his brother, if he were walking on the other side of the road. Harry often thought about Jason, but couldn't bring himself to contact him. What would they talk about anyway? Harry started to put his thoughts in order. I need a list, his mind shouted. He grabbed a pad of paper and began to write: How to survive this crisis, think like an army man.

The list, he carefully wrote, went on to over a hundred and twenty items, including medical items, in case of emergency. When Harry finished, Aida emerged, her deep sleep finally coming to an end. She was still in her nightclothes and still had her hairnet on her head.. To be honest, the couple had ceased to be attracted to each other many years ago. They took each other for granted. They could still argue like cats and dogs, but somehow always managed to make up. In the past it would be with a cuddle, or something even more intimate, but in recent years, they sidestepped even this. Harry would simmer and sulk, while Aida kept to herself and found ways to stay out of Harry's way, retreating to their vegetable garden, which in truth was minuscule and insignificant.

"What ya doing Harry?" Aida demanded, not even wishing him a good morning greeting of any kind.

"What does it look like?" Harry snapped back, not even

affording her a quick glance. "You aren't writing one of your lists, off to the shops are ya?" Aida said shuffling about, while thinking what to have for breakfast.

"There's this pandemic," Harry said earnestly, his eyes lit up. "Don't ya know? We need to get stocked up. I have calculated the shops will run out of food."

"Pan what...?" Aida demanded, a quizzical look on her face.

"You heard me," Harry sighed. "A pandemic - a virus spreading round the world, came from China where people eat rats, or so I read."

"People eating rats?" Aida sighed. "Why in God's name would they do that? Don't they have proper food?"

"Yeah well," said Harry, drawing in a deep breath. "Now we need to stock up. Can't take any unnecessary risks that will leave us short. We are in a survival situation. You get me Aida?"

"If you say so Harry. Doubtless you know best, but will our pensions cover all this food, you are going to buy?"

"I put enough money aside for a rainy day and this Aida, if you have been following the news is a critical moment that needs careful planning for the unexpected."

"I hope you have put my favourite fruit cake on the list and jaffa cakes, too."

"Listen Aida, jaffa cakes ain't going to keep you alive, where a tin of Fray Bentos might."

"Listen Harry," Aida said, shaking her head, "You're not in the army now and we are not at war."

"You keep telling me that," answered Harry, wagging his finger in Aida's face. "But my army training tells me to be prepared for any eventuality."

"Really Harry," mused Aida. "Ya never change, we will still be able to go to McDonalds. I love a Big Mac and, of course, you'd never take me to a restaurant."

Harry didn't bother to respond. The idea of isolating with Aida was going to prove burdensome, despite all those years of being married to her. Aida poured herself a coffee and put two chunky pieces of bread in the toaster as Harry reflected and continued to scribble away, his list getting longer and longer by the second. Aida imagined him coming home with a lorry load. Harry had this eager expression on his face, a look she was familiar with, and when he was like this, there was no turning back, no reasoning. He had always been a bit of a doomsayer. According to him, an asteroid was heading for earth or the country was going to be overrun by immigrants, who would take everybody's jobs, spreading disease and pestilence along the way. Harry believed this was the gospel truth

Aida blamed the newspapers he read. His favourite newspaper said as much, it was full of doom and sensational impending disasters. Yes, Harry was like this, always had been. He was scared and, yes, it was him who'd stopped her from having a baby, presenting a list of risks and reasons why not, while her heart yearned for a child. What kind of father would he have been anyway? He was inflexible and rigid and, yes, he was selfish. Bill, his brother, had said as much and apparently he'd always been like this. Maybe in his old age, she thought, he was getting worse and worse.

Once Harry completed his list and, after he'd painstakingly reviewed it several times, he looked at his watch and set off, hardly saying goodbye to Aida, who was left munching her toast, by herself. She heard him revving up the car, and speeding down their street, off on his mission to buy a survival kit of food that would see them through. A few thoughts flashed through her mind, perhaps in his haste Harry had overlooked certain practical considerations. Harry put on the radio - it was mostly local news, nothing of note.

The largest supermarket was about a ten-minute drive, depending on the traffic. At one point Harry angrily beeped his horn at some children, who kicked their football along the road by mistake. Harry was only a few minutes from the supermarket, when suddenly his car started to make noises, squealing like a banshee, the sound emanating from under the bonnet. Harry cursed and banged his fists on the steering wheel. When he stepped out of the car, he could smell something was not right. He reached for a small mobile phone kept in his jacket pocket. Suddenly, the cold realization hit him, it wasn't there. Aida had planned to wash his jacket and had emptied all his pockets. Harry saw a cyclist and signalled to him that he needed some assistance. The cyclist duly slowed down. "I am so sorry, but I need some help," Harry said in a breathy voice. "You happen to have a phone on you?" Harry said in a breathy voice. The cyclist had a small backpack and reached into it, taking out a phone.

"My car has broken down," explained Harry. "I need to call a garage."

"Look, why not try this garage," the cyclist said, flicking through his contacts. "I used it once myself, they do a good job,"

"Yes, okay, thanks for your help" Harry said, taking the phone and putting it to his ear.

"Gilbertson's garage," answered a woman cheerily. "How can I help you?"

"Yes, my name is Harry Hoarder and my car has broken down and I was wondering if you could send somebody to fix it. It is most urgent."

"I understand, sir, but our breakdown recovery service is busy. There was a big accident a short while ago, but, if you can wait a few hours, somebody will come and look at your problem." Harry grimaced, but didn't have many options.

He was somewhat in the middle of nowhere, without his phone and the cyclist looked eager to be on his way. Grudgingly, Harry gave the woman, details of his car's location, hung up, then thanked the cyclist. So, began a long wait for the recovery service to arrive. Harry was hungry and didn't even have anything much to occupy himself during the long wait. Time passed slowly. At one point, he even thought there was a van coming to his aid, but it proved a false hope.

He was about to give up, maybe flag down another person, when a truck with Gilbertson's Garage Repairs in large letters, drove slowly towards him.

"Thank God," Harry exclaimed. "I'm so happy to see you. I thought you'd never come."

A man wearing green overalls and a cap with the Gilbertson's logo got out of the truck. "What's the problem, Mate?" he asked, peering at Harry through slit eyes.

"The car started making squealy noises, then broke down," Harry explained with a deep sigh.

"Best have a look at it" the mechanic replied, walking over to Harry's stricken car. It didn't take the mechanic long to locate the problem. The serpentine belt had snapped.

"Have you had this car a long time, it looks pretty old?" asked the mechanic. Harry had to admit, it was an old car and he should have replaced it.

"This car is as good as scrap," sighed the mechanic. "Come to our garage and we can sort you out a replacement, but you are going to have to consider buying a new car. This one has had it." Harry cursed silently, but heeded the mechanic's advice.

When they reached the garage, Harry was shown a vehicle that could replace his broken auto. He was also given a hefty bill for the job of removing his car from the side of the road and for the use of a replacement car. But, to Harry, what was worse was that he'd lost time, valuable time – time he could have spent getting in all that food and other vital provisions to see him and Aida through the coming pandemic.

Gritting his teeth, he paid the bill and left the garage in the replacement car. He soon found his way to the giant supermarket. There was an unusual number of cars parked in the lot and people milling about the entrance to the store, but Harry was not deterred. He walked in a determined fashion and grabbed a supermarket trolley. As he approached the entrance, he noticed people wheeling their trolleys out, all overflowing with products, One woman in particular seemed to have a mountain of toilet rolls. What does she have? Harry asked himself. A football team living with her. Because of all the shoppers, there was a wait before Harry could even enter the supermarket. Suddenly, a new dreadful thought struck him, his list - his precious list was on the dashboard of his car. He'd taken it out to look over again and forgotten to put it back in his pocket. His list, his mind cursed several times, he'd managed to mislay his list! The day couldn't get any worse, or could it? He told himself to keep cool, not to fret, all those methods, he'd learned, while in the army about staying in control.

He thought about the first two items on the list – toilet paper and tea bags. His first task was to find the aisle with toilet paper. Walking down the aisles, he finally found the one where the toilet rolls could be found. He tried to push his trolley down the aisle, but it was crowded. It seemed like a cluster of people had beaten him to it and were grabbing at packets of toilet paper with an unnatural eagerness – a sight Harry had never experienced in his long life.

Sighing, he knew he would have to bide his time. But when his chance arrived, there was only a limited choice left. He found a few rolls of pink toilet paper which he calculated would last only days rather than weeks. But that was all there was. He took the two remaining packets, despite the fact, that an old lady who stood behind him would leave empty-handed. Many of the shelves in the supermarket looked like they had been ravaged by rampaging panic buyers, in truth somewhat like himself. His trolley, even after spending quite a lengthy time in the supermarket, seemed horribly threadbare. Other people had taken all the long-lasting food and cans, leaving terrible choices, which Harry was forced to buy. The shelves usually full of pasta had been stripped bare. Harry just gawped at the empty spaces where food would normally reside. All the packets of paracetamol were gone, had been snapped up hours ago, so the supermarket employee said in a cold detached way.

Harry joined the line of shoppers, who also had empty-looking trolleys. If not for the car problem, Harry thought he would have been fine - home hours ago. When it was his turn to pay, a rather miserable-looking cashier gave him a vague smile. All his goods were scanned and it was time for him to pay. He handed over his card. The cashier rammed it in the machine and tapped a few buttons and then shook her head.

"Is there a problem?" Harry asked, anxiously.

The cashier shrugged, "I am afraid there is, sir. There's a problem with your card, maybe it has expired. Harry looked at her in absolute shock.

"You are joking aren't you!" Harry exclaimed, his face getting paler and paler by the second. His world was collapsing. "Try again, won't you?"

The cashier sighed, "Not sure it will do any good, sir." She tapped again. "No, sir, there is nothing I can do, you will just have to put all the goods back."

There was nothing much Harry could say, no arguments he could put up, there was no way round the stark truth, he had to put each item back. The old lady who couldn't get hold of any toilet paper was delighted, when he placed the rolls he had claimed for himself back on the shelf. Some of the other items he'd taken were also gladly latched onto by desperate shoppers. Once he'd completed his depressing task of redistributing his goods, he trudged back outside to his car. When he arrived back at his house, he caught sight of Aida, staring out of the window, an anxious look on her face. He walked solemnly down the garden path, arms empty, his mind full of regrets.

"Where the hell have you been?" Aida demanded, as he stepped inside their house. She glared at him and added, "You have been hours." Harry felt ashamed and awkward.

"First the car went," Harry groaned, "and broke down. Next my card wouldn't work at the supermarket." Aida held up a letter the bank had sent months before, which Harry had forgotten about, as it had gathered dust.

"I was going to ask you about your card before you left, Harry, but you stormed out of the house. And, I couldn't call you because you left your phone here, too."

"Yes Aida," said Harry, downcast. "I know, and the car cost me a fortune."

"So what are we going to do about food, Harry?" Aida asked, peering into her husband's eyes, expecting answers.

"Well," said Harry, drawing in a sharp breath. "We will just have to hope I succeed tomorrow, where I failed today."

Aida was far from satisfied by Harry's response. In her eyes he had failed. The two of them spent a painful evening barely talking to one another. When he went the next day expectantly to the supermarket, the shelves had been barely replenished. One shopper had quipped to Harry, "you are too late mate, everything has been snapped up by a load of hoarders." Harry had grimly smiled. The Hoarder's supplies were horribly short. When Harry returned to Aida, she looked with disgust at the meagre amount of supplies he had managed to acquire. She screamed at him to leave the house and not return until he had acquired enough food to see them through, this impending crisis. It was a hopeless task.

January 16, 3:33 PM

Shannon Pratuch

Baby dear
Let us lie down
Just for a moment

Lawnmower drones
Smell of cut grass
Warming in the April air
A bee visits to say hello
Hello hello hello

Dig your toes into
The grass the earth
You will return far too
Early than I am ready
My living heart

Silent night, lonely night

Linda Watkins

THE YOUNG MAN stood by the window gazing down at the street below. His face was like a blank page, waiting for someone, anyone, to write something on it.

Empty. The street was dead.

Sighing, he turned from the window and made his way over to the kitchen pantry. There was just enough light left to see inside. The power had gone off ten days before and he'd given up hope that it would go back on anytime soon. He only had one flashlight and knew he had to conserve the few batteries he had left.

Gazing at the half-empty shelves, he once again counted. Five cans of beans, three cans of chopped tomatoes, a can of mushroom soup, a one pound bag of brown rice, a six pack of Coke with one can missing, a bag of Fritos, a box of Rice-A-Roni, and a one pound package of pasta. Not much left. He'd soon have to go out foraging. It was a thought he didn't want to entertain, but it was that or starve to death.

Death, he thought. A concept he was now all too familiar with.

He stared at his meagre supplies, shaking his head. When the electricity died, he'd had to eat everything in the refrigerator first and he'd cursed the fact that it was summer. If it had been winter, he could have put some of the frozen stuff outside on the fire escape so it would last longer. But that was his luck – all bad.

He decided he'd eat a half-can of beans for dinner, cold. He wished his stove had been powered by gas, but it wasn't. He'd always prided himself on his all-electric kitchen. Now, he laughed at his foolishness.

Tears welled in his eyes as he sat on arm of the living room sofa. How irresponsible they'd all been. He wished now he could turn back the clock and start over. How differently he'd do things. He thought about his mom, his dad, his sister – all gone because of his disdain for the truth – because of his conceit.

He wiped away a tear that was sliding down his cheek. He was only twenty-two for Christ's sake! Barely a man. He had his whole life ahead of him. But what kind of life would it be now? Everyone he loved was gone – everyone he knew was gone. Fuck it, for all he knew there was no one else left at all!

He gazed at his iPad sitting silently on the coffee table. It was useless now. No power and the Internet had crashed weeks ago anyway. If there were anyone left in this city, he had no way to reach out to them.

Suddenly, he froze, eyes wide with surprise. Was that a sound coming from the street outside?

A car? Or was he just hallucinating?

Quickly, he ran to the window, heart pounding. A truck was slowly making its way down the street. It was the first vehicle he'd seen in days. Clumsily, he struggled with the window lock, finally pushing it open.

"Hey!" he yelled, waving his arms madly. "Up here! Hey! Stop!"

But the truck lumbered on.

Furious, he slammed the window shut. He grabbed his jacket and headed for the door that led to the fire escape. Maybe if he hurried, he could catch up to the truck.

As he dashed down the steps, he tried to remember the last time he'd seen another human. Was it one week or two? He'd tried all the apartments in his complex more than once, but no one answered when he knocked. Most, he knew, had left town before the virus caught hold, moving to less congested parts of the country. But he'd stayed. After all, he was young and everybody said the disease was mostly fatal to the old and those with compromised immune systems.

An almost hysterical chuckle escaped from his throat when he thought about that. His sister was only eighteen and she'd died. She wasn't old and didn't have cancer or anything like that. No, the supposedly wise pundits were wrong. This virus didn't care what age you were or how healthy you were. It just jumped from person to person like some sort of demented grasshopper. And without knowing, he'd helped it along.

That thought almost paralyzed him. He took a deep breath. If he froze now, his last hope might slip away. Forcing himself, he continued down the steep stairs. But despite his resolve, he couldn't turn off his mind.

The authorities had warned everyone. Stay inside they said. Practice social distancing. But he hadn't listened. He wasn't going to change his lifestyle because of a bug like the flu. No, he'd kept hanging with his friends, going to bars that stayed open despite the shut-down order, making out with girls he hardly knew.

And, as a result, he'd gotten sick – a low-grade fever, some coughing, but it wasn't bad. It didn't stop him from going to Sunday dinner at his parents' place.

He stifled a sob when he thought about his foolishness. He'd infected them all that night. Killed them. He'd murdered them with hugs and handshakes. Murdered them with his carelessness and his love.

Shaking off his despair, he continued rushing down the fire escape stairs, leaping off the bottom step to the pavement. Gazing down the street, he could still see the truck – just a block and a half ahead of him.

He ran toward it, waving his arms and screaming.

"Help!" he cried. "I'm all alone! Help! Please, don't leave me here!"

The truck stopped.

A ray of hope blossomed in the young man's heart.

A middle-aged man wearing a Red Sox ball cap stuck his head out the window and stared at him.

"Hey you," the driver yelled. "I recognize you. You're Bill Thompson's kid. You're the piece of shit who gave it to my niece, Kaitlin."

The young man stopped running. Kaitlin? Did he know a Kaitlin? He searched his memory but all he could come up with was a girl he'd met one night at one of the clubs. Long blonde hair, big blue eyes. Her name escaped him – was it Kathy, Katie, Kaitlin? He couldn't remember for sure. They'd had sex that night in the backseat of his car in the parking lot. A few days later he'd woken up with a cough. Had he given it to her that night? Had his wet kisses sealed her death warrant? Or, had she given it to him? He didn't know and had to admit he didn't really care. They were both to blame – both of them, so sure of their own immortality – their youth – their sense of invincibility – all proved false by one fucking little germ.

As these thoughts raced across his mind, the truck driver continued to watch him silently, waiting.

"Please," the young man begged, falling to his knees as if in prayer. "I didn't mean it. I didn't know. Please help me."

The man in the truck laughed. "You didn't know? Christ, did you live in a cave? You're an infector! Selfish bastard! Thought nothing could touch you? Well, what do you think now? You won't die of the freaking bug, but you will die, won't you? Die of desperation – die of loneliness."

The young man felt hot tears stain his cheeks.

"Please … I didn't mean it … please!"

The driver stared at him for a moment as if perhaps he were having second thoughts. Then he spat on the ground, pulled his head back inside, and put the truck in gear. He took off down the road then turned the corner fast, tires squealing, as if he couldn't wait to get as far from this city as possible.

"Please," the young man whispered even though there was no one left to hear. "Don't leave me here alone. I can't take it much longer."

But the truck was gone and, once again, the street was deserted.

The young man slowly got to his feet and, head bowed, began walking back to his apartment.

The sun was setting. It was time to open that can of beans.

My little apocalypse

Christopher T Dabrowski

Snow covered neighbourhood, as far as the eye can see. Reality mantled frosty, ominous silence. It was too quiet, for too long it has lasted. I felt it subcutaneously – this calm before the storm, it is about to begin, the next end of the world will happen.

I was not wrong. Darkness came. Earth tremors came.

Black of the sky cut through luminous colours. Snow rotated rising to the heavens.

The world turned upside down. Literally… the sky at the bottom, the ground at the top.

Suddenly it settled down.

When snow fell I saw an enormous eye at the sky. On the horizon of events, large, deformed tooth grinned. In a moment a creature drifted away.

Phew, it didn't devour me!

This is what the apocalypse in a decorative sphere with snow looked like.

My Small Green Prayers

Margot Henderson

Oh there are some days
when I can barely summon
the energy to take a breath.

I feel so full of sorrow and despair
at all the suffering on this precious Earth
grieving the pointless cruelty and death.

I feel hopeless, helpless, overwhelmed
wondering what is the point of anything
feeling incapable of rising with the spring.

In those moments, the only place
where I feel calmed
is in the refuge of my garden.

My body soothed and softening
when I hear the blackbird sing,
drawing the air and sunlight in
bringing the buds to blossom on the stem.

I feel the world come to life again
I draw another breath
and plant my small green prayers in the earth.

We

Adele C. Geraghty

Outside, the air is crisp and cool with the promise of poison
A possible touch, brush, nudge, ready to determine death
from a smile, a sigh, a friendly wave within a step, too close!
We've closed the door, leaving risk outside. This is lockdown.

Expecting an apocalypse, shops empty in hours.
Food is left outside our door by unknown volunteers.
I used to volunteer. I should be distributing with them.
But, you and I are high risk. We thank them behind our masks.

Calmly, each day our eyes ask each other,
Are you holding up? Are we alright? And as always
'Yes! I'm fine! We're fine!' 'We will survive'.
Then we watch the news. Each night animals are frolicking.

In vacant streets across the globe, penguins, goats, elephants.
Am I a traitor to my species, when my heart skips with the beauty
of their reclamation, wishing it might never stop? Willing a new age?
I cup, lovingly, your hands in mine, feeling their tender strangeness.

Your bones, a fretwork of birds, nesting beneath translucent skin,
which dips and rises, presenting its depths of infinite, rhythmic
    rainbow, of life in situ,
seemingly and deceptively endless. When did your hands become
    so fragile?
Perhaps in the missing breath of time, when I began breathing
    with difficulty.

Or when I began to stop more frequently when we walked. When do we say
enough? Will we know when it's time and open the door, smiling as I shelter
your hand and you support my fragile hip, facing a forever of completing each
others' sentences, breathing the crisp, cool air outside?

FUNNY STUFF IN LOCKDOWN

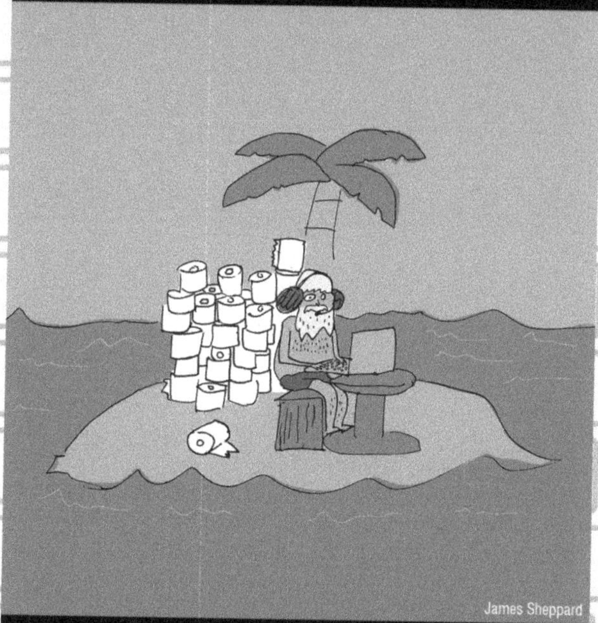

Neal Zetter, Francis H Powell, NZ, Peter Finch, Dom Conlon, Coral Rumble, Alan Durant, Professor Elemental, Ian McPherson

Clear Out the Shed

Neal Zetter

Rediscover stuff forgotten
Busted, broken, dusty, rotten
Boredom hit a new rock bottom?
"Let's clear out the shed"

Didn't know such junk existed
Scrap and crap piles all z-listed
It's a task to be resisted
"Let's clear out the shed"

"Let's clear out the shed"
"Let's clear out the shed"
Much prefer to eat my head
"Let's clear out the shed"

Never was one for spring cleaning
Who cares if this place is gleaming?
Tear your hair out then start screaming
"Let's clear out the shed"

Bike bits, wallpaper and paint pots
Plugs, rugs, cracked mugs, I don't know what
Chipped tiles, lino - bin the whole lot
"Let's clear out the shed"

"Let's clear out the shed"
"Let's clear out the shed"
Rather shoot myself instead
"Let's clear out the shed"

It's a task I've not requested
Mixing with the rat-infested
Have to get myself blood-tested
"Let's clear out the shed"

Garbage? What a huge selection
Mouldy mattress for rejection
Condoms unfit for protection
"Let's clear out the shed"

"Let's clear out the shed"
"Let's clear out the shed"
Find a body, long since dead
"Let's clear out the shed"

"Let's clear out the shed"
"Let's clear out the shed"
What's the job that you most dread?
"Let's clear out the shed"

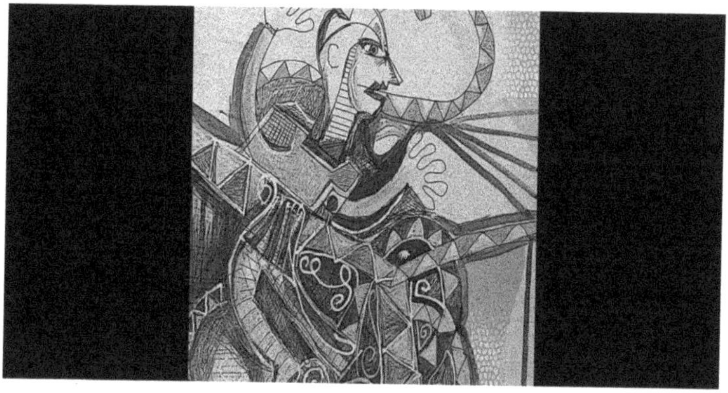

Confused Poet.com

Francis H Powell

Oh schizophrenic poet,
do you wonder who you are?
As the world keeps turning around
can your true identity be found
bamboozling inordinate shapes and sounds
One day you are wandering lonely as a cloud
then you're a part of some beatnik crowd,
just standing there silent but proud
then Doctor Seuss on a roller coaster
nonsense reigns in your head
you steal some words from a Shakespeare sonnet
shooting across the sky like a lyrical comet
The next day your words are both meaningful and divine
a spiritual guru getting drunk on rhyme
A poetical *Conquistador*, lost on the way
A post modern, neo-classical romantic caught in the fray
With words of beauty or lines of thorns
a poem springs up like the break of dawn

Are you the master of your fate
Are things all falling apart in your wake
You wake up all *Coleridge* in Xanadu
Go sleep with Sylvia Plath on your pillow
The Moon and the yew tree are haunting you so
A morning song in your mind as you walk down the road
Then you are struck by some lines of John Milton
Paradise is lost with a glass of port and some stilton
There's Virginia Wolf winding the hours all down
but my poems will never keep the wolf from the door
as bills keep on mounting, falling to the floor
and there's Ezra the anti-capitalist poet
selling England by the pound
and you invited John Keats if only he could come round
and traces of Lord Byron's melancholia
all of this can to be found slumped on your sofa
There's scattered papers on the floor
searching for your wanton soul, more and more
We should praise these Gods of a lyrical meter
touched by the sober tenderness of Sackville-West Vita
Open your doors to Jim Morrison world
his sharp mind and vision unfurled
absorbed and lost, an audience with a sacred druid
ancient verse like milk and honey so fluid,
one day you are Jekyll and then you are Hyde
one day the groom another day the bride
words stretched about like a Jim Carey face
juggling words like a basket case
a split personality with pen and ink
Poetry therapy with a poetical shrink.

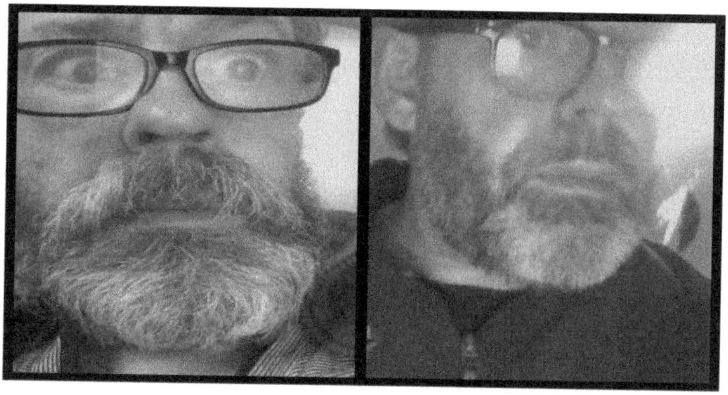

Rough Beard, Smooth Beard

Francis H Powell

Rough beard

I have a beard, a long grey beard
it's bristly itchy, most untoward
beyond all doubt and reason
I look like an ancient grizzled seaman
Call me Ahab or Nemo or Robinson Crusoe
or perhaps fungus face, will do so
Am I Sigmund Freud gone wild
or Charles Darwin, all beguiled
or George the fifth in all his glory
or a just a wanderer with a story
perhaps Poseidon, less a trident holding
Stuck on the land, bad tempered and moody
Socrates philosophically floundering
Will I end up like Rasputin
without the love of a Russian Queen
Am I just a beardy weirdy beatnik style?
Allan Ginsberg with a smile

Smooth beard

Before my beard was nicely groomed
all spic and span, finely attuned
not like a prehistoric man's,
it was cut and shaped with careful hands
I went to a barbers, not many months before
I looked much better, to be sure
In reflection, thinking back
I was quite respectable then
a paradigm amongst men
but now it can't be denied
I'm a castaway all cockeyed
I just stopped shaving,
it was labour-saving
Now I dare not look full in the mirror
to see my unkempt state
when will the barbers reopen
put a razor to my chin
wrestle my bristles back to normality
a makeover to shake off my fictional abnormality

Covid-19: Pavement Strategy

Neal Zetter

What's your pavement strategy?

Are you a **Lefter?**
Ever sticking
to the extreme
left-hand side
of the street

Or a **Righter?**
Keenly hugging
the opposite
right-hand flank

Or a **Middler?**
Cautiously...
stepping...
into spaces...
created by...
the above two...

Or a **Zig-zagger?**
Cleverly navigating any new gaps
as they appear

Or a **Roader?**
Relentlessly treading Tarmac
carefully dodging passing cars

Or are you a **Killer?**
A selfish w@$*er ignoring EVERY rule
Whose strategy is...
To have no strategy at all

What's your pavement strategy?

Our Mad House

Francis H Powell

OH calamity Ken, has been at it again
swinging his hips, climbing Big Ben
Then there's the lovely, most wonderful Dora,
she'll burst out crying, if you ignore her,
just back from the wonder island of Bora Bora
where life is just a game, ask any explorer

Terror boy Terry has plenty to eat
he can juggle with oranges
and his ration of meat
His sister Samantha is sat by the telly
and Mother Martina collapsed in a heap
Father Theodore is keeping them sane
as he tries to plant cabbages out in the rain
With the heat of the day, the children do sway
trying to cast their boredom away
But don't come round to our madhouse today
it is not allowed anyway

Fun boy Philip is doing a dance
with his uncles and cousins and some of his aunts
Scallywag Stephen is running on gas
while that Father McCrockingdale is saying his mass
Horrible Henry is breaking up houses
Norman Wilkins thinks he's Johann Strauss
Millington Milly is picking daisies
while Jeremy Jones is going crazy

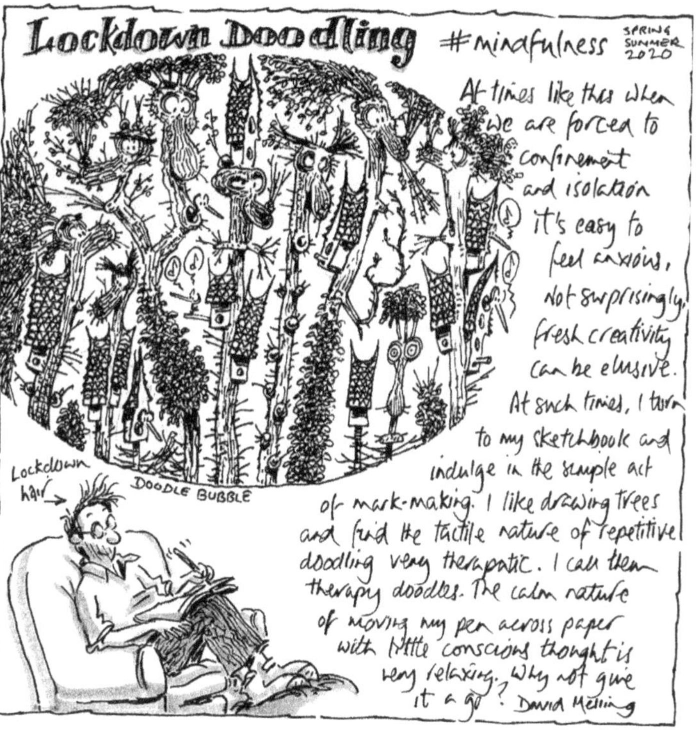
Lockdown Doodling
#mindfulness
SPRING
SUMMER
2020
At times like this when we are forced to confinement and isolation it's easy to feel anxious, not surprisingly, fresh creativity can be elusive. At such times, I turn to my sketchbook and indulge in the simple act of mark-making. I like drawing trees and find the tactile nature of repetitive doodling very therapeutic. I call them therapy doodles. The calm nature of moving my pen across paper with little conscious thought is very relaxing. Why not give it a go? David Melling
Lockdown hair
DOODLE BUBBLE

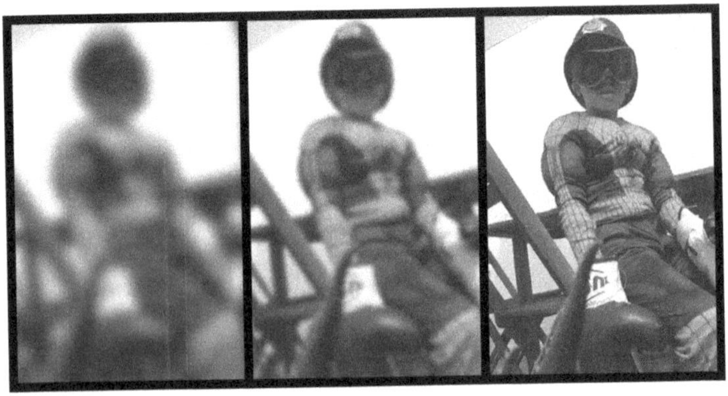

My Quirky Son

Francis H Powell

My son has his quirky ways
asks for garlic bread for breakfast
He has be known to ask for the strangest dishes
it hard to keep up with all his wishes
porridge and egg bread are his favourite food
Weetabix, but no milk when he's in the mood
All is smothered in ketchup and mayonnaise
it's hard to put a stop to this unhealthy phase
He wants a grass snake for a pet
but what would happen if it needs a vet
His head is often deep in cartoons
I am worried by the world that he consumes
He is always lucky finding money
that people have dropped on their way
he could find treasure in a cave
or ride to America surfing a wave
Romance on the TV just makes him squirm
his face shrivels up, like a withered up worm

He dresses up in strange clothing combinations
but you can only laugh at his unusual aberrations.

Summer clothes in winter
and winter clothes in summer
hitting with drum sticks
like an over hyped up drummer
Then there are all his science experiments
and those meteorites he's collected
Ready for sport at half past six on a Sunday morning
to spring into action barely yawning
He always has short-lived obsessions
his ever changing preoccupations
One week football catches his attention
the next week it barely gets a mention.

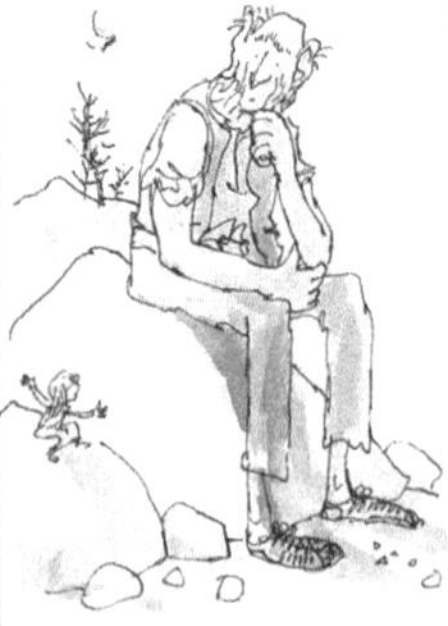

The Making of Roald Dahl

Peter Finch

Richard Diddley, Singer
Richy Dosher, Schwama Maker
Ricky Doodle, Echo Winner
Ricko Ditcher, Lifetime Drinker
R.S Dinas, Queen Street Statue
Ronnie Dickens, Juggler
Ron Dawkins, Man of the Woods
Ronald Davies, Pork Butcher
Ronald Dawes, Confectioner
Ronald Drift, Handyperson
Ronald Dill, Brakeman
Reginald Dosanquest, TV Reporter
Reggie Darling, Cutter of Coal
Rennie Derringer, Industrial Chemist
Rollie Dark, Canton Magician
Roland Desketh, Government Agent
Roland Delwydd, Hillside Farmer
Roland Dafis, Chapel Decorator

Ronal Despor, Rodent Remover
Roland Dal, Ship Stay Manufacturer
Roland Dil, Iron Moulder
Roland Doll, Airline Pilot
Roland Dell, Pencil Maker
Roland Barthes, Philosopher
Roland Corona, Pop Inflator
Roland Singer, Mussleman
Reggie Dahl, Gunrunner
Roland Dahl, Awdur
Roald Dahl, BFG

Small World

Dom Conlon

I've got a gym inside my kitchen
And the seaside's in my room
The world has shrunk so blooming much
That I can touch the moon.

The hallway is the motorway
I use to see my dad,
But no-one checks my licence card
So that part's not so bad.

I flush the loo (now that's the train)
Whilst chatting to our Jack,
I take a ticket from the roll—
It's good for there and back.

We've had to change the clocks to suit
The way the world's so small
Or else I'd be the fastest kid
Gold medals? Got them all!

So now I say I've travelled well
Now that the world is small
But that gym inside my kitchen
Isn't getting used at all.

I won't talk about Corona

Coral Rumble

I'd like to talk to you today
As I'm feeling like a loner,
I'll talk about most anything,
But not about Corona.
I'll talk about my aunty
And how she is a moaner,
I'll talk about my grandma
And how I wish you'd known her,
I'll talk about my brother
Who's always been a roamer,
I'll talk about my cousin,
How I really need to phone her,
I'll talk about my neighbor
And the ladder I might loan her,
I'l talk about smooth dolphins
And how they run on sonar,
I'll talk about my frisky horse–
You wouldn't want to own her,
I'll talk about aerobics
How it really makes me groan(er),
I'll talk about my editor and
The new work that I've shown her,
I'll talk about most anything,
BUT NOT ABOUT CORONA!

(Unlike Me They Want to Be) Too Close to You

Alan Durant

Today my sense of humour has shrivelled
to the size of a crumpled tissue tossed in a wastepaper bin;
If I see one more person on my usually solitary way through the woods

those two women, for example, with an older man puffing behind them,
or that family out walking their dog,
or the woman with five dogs on an ever extending lead,
or the couple in full fell hiking gear,

then I'll throw something,
a barbed remark probably about government rules
on social distancing when exercising during the coronavirus pandemic.

But then I see them:
cluster upon cluster of bluebells,
their lilac heads hanging as if preparing for a group nod,
their silence clamorous in my heart.

Who cares that they are barely centimetres apart,
never mind the required two metres,
or that they are out in such numbers
that this thicket could be renamed Bluebell Wood?

This is a day for solitude not sharing;
I like people well enough in general,
but even those I love I wouldn't want to be here now
with their chattering, ideas, opinions and observations.

No, let the birds, sensibly isolated at the top of their trees,
do the talking, giving voice to whatever it is that concerns
birds at this Spring time of year -

worms, I guess, and finding a mate,
or wondering perhaps, with a mite of irritation,
why it is that human beings suddenly appear every time
their loved one is near.

The Difficulties of Homeschooling an Orangutan

Professor Elemental

At first we both liked the challenge
I made a jungle for him in the lounge
Book-cases were trees
So was the settee
Added taxidermied birds that I found

But by lunchtime on day 2, all was chaos
Sticky rinds and fruit stains on the curtains
The world was unbalanced
I was up to the challenge
But poor Geoffrey looked on, uncertain

Day three, I hid under a table
He raged for the entire duration
It's inadvisable at best
To put apes to the test
Let alone teach algebraic equations

But over the months, I felt lucky
Whether we laughed or we cried
Cosy cuddled in covers
At least we have each other
Looking out at the world from inside

After months of confinement we're free
No more fights or home-made lessons
Geoffrey's back in the trees
I'm and I'm sat back in peace
Appreciating the teaching profession.

Hardly a fit subject for levity – Episode 11

Ian McPherson

One man.
A shed.
Three tiny nonagenarian aunts.

For once I was feeling pretty chipper. Is that the right word? Chipper? Thing is, I felt good. It was one of those balmy summer days. The Telefunken sat, silent as a memory, in the corner. No aunts as far as the ear could hear. The only sound –

Okay. Let me fess up here. I was reading a first edition copy of Sloot. I know, I know. I wrote it. So? I hadn't actually read it. And I'll be quite honest. It's a hoot. Anyway, there I was, twelve weeks into the deadliest virus the world has ever known, sitting alone in the shed reading my own work and hooting with life-affirming joy. I turned to page two, still hooting, although I wasn't actually reading at the time. I was mid-sentence. One half read, one half still to go. Check it out. But not now. God it was funny. Both bits. Did I say hoot? As in *Sloot* is a comploot hoot? I was –

But wait. A grunting noise outside. More of a triple grunt. I closed the book and secreted it under another copy of *Sloot*. It was the only thing on the desk. Okay okay. Fess up time again. I'd bought a box. Good thing too, because it certainly bears rereading. So. *Sloot* under *Sloot*. Triple grunt. I went over and opened the –

'Howaya, Een. It's only us. Give us a hand here or we'll bleedin' burst you. Only joshin. Now this bag, which totally blocks us from view – look over the top –'

'– Peekaboo! –'

'– is a pile of books from our clearout. Hoick it inside and we'll explain everyting.'

I did as requested, managing to block, in so doing, a view of both *Sloots*. Self-publicity has never been my style.

'So, ladies,' I said, returning to my seat and using double-*Sloot* as an arm rest, 'explain away. You have the floor. Alternatively, pray be seated. You have the armchair.'

As you can probably tell, I was still feeling a bit light-headed from my reading – *Sloot*, as you'll recall, bottom copy – and may have had to stifle a slightly high-pitched giggle at the memory. Funny stuff.

'Right, Een. We are now happily ensconced. And here's our tinking. In the early seventeent century, at the height of whatever plague was fashionable at the time, the playwright William Shakespeare was confined to his lodgings for the durayshing.'

'There was only one book in the house.'

'Wait for it! "The Compleat Works of William Shakespeare".'

'When they finally popped in to tell him it was safe to go out, they found him laughing hysterically at the final couplet of Otello's last speech. Which is not, in most productions of the play in the intervening centuries, played for laughs.'

'There's actually a reference to the same play on page 57 of your breakout novel, "Sloot". You don't happen to have a copy on the premises?'

'Sadly no, ladies.'

'Probly just as well, Een. They carted old Will out of there and, in spite of writing several smash hit plays and being feted the lengt and bret of the West End, he was never the same since.'

'Of course they didn't have mental healt in those days. You just picked yourself up, adjusted your codpiece, and got on wit it.'

'If, heaven forfend, the same ting happened to you, Een –'

'Well that's hardly likely, is it?' I may have tittered as I said it, which wasn't my intention, but I'm pretty sure they didn't notice.

'Which is why we've brought you some of our vast library for your delectayshing and delight.'

'Interesting point, Een. The age of book burning is back. Big time. If you don't like it, or the autor ruffles your ego, burn it.'

'Gas, isn't it? We've cancelled our log deliveries for the next two years.'

'Settle down, ladies. You don't have a log fire.'

'Just as well we cancelled then.'

'Anyway, where were we?'

'Delectation, as I recall. And delight.'

'Thing is, Een, we've been clearing out our bookshelves. And this'll kill you. Not literously, so relax. Ready?'

"Tinking outside the Trousers", a self-help book for the intelligent male, and the perfect antidote to "Let your Penis do the Talking".'

'Don't know why we had it in the first place.'

'Burn it.'

'We'll ignore that. Right. Jane Austing's only crime triller.'

'I didn't know she'd written one.'

'Poor sales, Een. It's not a good idea to give the who dunnit persing away in the title.'

BEAT. SIGH.

'And the title was?'

"Reader, I Murdered Him". Oh, you'll like this one. "Great Eyebrows in History". Did you know all the great eyebrows are male? John Knox, he of the barbed wire underpants. Wing Commander Victor don't-call-me-Victoria Cross. His were requisitioned for the war effort, Een. Launch pads for spitfires.'

'And finally, you're going to love this – an uncorrected proof of the latest Toby Smyrke.'

'Really?'

'Uh oh. No love lost there, we see. Professional jealousy, peut-être?'

'Certainly not.'

'We should perhaps explain for the casual voyeur –'

'Not voyeur, Dottie. You can't see it and there's no rude bits. Sorry, where was I?'

(COLD) 'Tobias Smyrke.'

'Oh, Tobias now, is it? You really don't like him, do you? Tobias Smyrke, Autor, shortlisted for that big book award wit "Aranchophilia".'

'Bloody incomprehensible, frankly.'

'Spider's web structure, Een. Bet you wish you'd tought of it first.'

'Yeh. Right.'

'Anyway, his latest, due to hit the lack of shelves – a glancing reference to the plague stroke virus of 2020 there, Een – weighs in at 12 hundred and 46 pages.'

'Jesus. Never use one small word when twelve big ones will do.'

'It's a one-word novel.'

(SIGH) 'Of course it is.'

'Title?'

'Don't tell me. "word". Lower case on the w.'

'Precisually so.'

'Toby Smyrke. "The novel is dead. I should know, I killed it."' And here's you starting a new one.'

'There's your title. "Dodo". Get it?'

'Yes, I get it.'

'But Toby's pleasing flatulence brings us to your maiden effort at the novel form, Een, in which you tried your hand at an Irish "War and Peace".'

'Aldough you wouldn't know that from the title.'

'"The Nut House".'

'On you go, Een. We've brought popcorn.'

***

I had just placed the job advertisement in the window and was chopping ingredients for the day's special when the phone rang.

'Nut House?' I said. 'No, no. It's a common mistake, Doctor. This is the vegetarian restaurant of the same name.'

No sooner had I put the phone down and got back to work than the door burst open and in burst a man with a gun. That's two bursts in one sentence, but the word has a certain onomatopoeic quality and it suited both door and man. So. Door. Man with gun. Double burst.

He pointed the gun at me in what I can only describe as an aggressive manner.

'Put the knife down,' he spat. 'And move away from the courgette. Now.'

My restaurant my rules I thought, but there was something in his tone which wouldn't be gainsaid. I did as he asked.

'If this is about the job,' I said, 'then I have to tell you you've got off to a very bad start. Look at those shoes. Filthy.'

'It's not about the job.'

'In that case,' I said, wiping my hands on my apron, 'what can I get you?'

I sincerely hoped he wasn't going to say 'Mmmn. Your special looks nice. Think I'll plump for that.' I have an unfortunate habit of chalking up the menu first, then getting down to the more protracted business of preparing and cooking. Call it aggressive marketing. At any rate, there it stood. 'Today's Special – Pizza Del Journo.'

'I'm not hungry,' he snapped. Still, I noted, brandishing the gun.

'Café Latte?' I said. 'Cappuccino? Americano? Espresso? Café Del Journo?'

I was starting to feel flamboyant in a Mediterranean sort of way, but he didn't seem impressed. His attention had been diverted by the sudden arrival of a veritable phalanx of cop cars in the street outside. Sirens blaring. Tyres squealing. Horns tooting. And encroaching on the cycle lane with apparent impunity. I was, however, pretty sanguine about the whole thing. This is the world we live in. Accept it or look elsewhere. My new acquaintance, on the other hand, was positively vexed.

'Jesus!'

He threw a table over – not, fortunately, one I'd already laid – crouched behind it and waggled his pistol. A tad provocative to my way of thinking, but I had other things to worry about. Not a single enquiry since I'd placed the job ad. I mean what is it with kids these days? Do they not want to work? I was also feeling a bit sensitive about the apparent lack of custom. Time, perhaps, to have a rethink on the price structure. As if that wasn't enough, I was still at the chopping, dicing, grating stage, when I should be simmering at the very least. My uninvited guest may have been above such mundane matters, but I had a business to run.

'Mind if I get on?' I said. And then, pointedly, 'I mean these dishes don't cook themselves.'

He seemed preoccupied with his own thoughts, so I took that as a yes. And as I diced the carrots, chopped the leeks and grated the Parmesan, I studied the back of his head. Orange bristles stood out from his neck like quills upon the fretful porpentine. The tension in his shoulder muscles was palpable. Now I don't wish to be melodramatic, but he really did look capable of inflicting serious injury on person or persons unknown. Diet, I thought. Too much raw meat. This is a typical vegetarian response, but it's a well-known fact: non-carnivores are far less likely to respond aggressively in any given situation; Hitler being the honourable exception to this particular rule.

And then it struck me. This aggression had nothing to do with diet. But of course! How could I have been so blind? Orange hair? Accent not a million miles from the Catholic quarter of Ballymena? I knew Ballymena well, having been drummed out of there on several occasions. Failure to wear bowler hat in public place. Accent likely to cause breach of peace. That sort of thing. But there I had it. The key to all his pent-up fury. His incandescent rage. And before I could stop myself I blurted my thoughts into words. 'For pity's sake put the gun down, lad. You're in Edinburgh now. And besides, the blessed war is over.'

Well that was a great relief. Momentarily.

'What the hell are you on about?' he all but shrieked. And then he got back to his ridiculous game with the police. One of whom was bellowing into a megaphone in a shocking display of inconsideration. Noise pollution? Karaoke by the back door I call it.

But I digress.

'Oh yes,' I said. 'The war ended some time back. Catholics and Protestants now live together in peace and harmony. Apart, obviously, from the odd ritual slaughter.'

The back of his head gave me a withering look.

'It's nothing to do with the war,' he snapped.

I was more than happy to correct him on this particular point.

'Ah, but that's where you're wrong, you see. It's a post traumatic stress type thing. The psychological inability to let seven hundred years of mindless brutality go. And you've got it, sonny. In spades.'

He said nothing. A helicopter was about to land on the roof opposite and it may have appealed to his boyish sense of wonder. At any rate he was transfixed by its perilous descent. But I was on a roll, so I sculpted a yam into peace symbols and developed my thesis anyway.

'Oh, we've all experienced the after effects of conflict,' I said. 'Take my tragic background, for instance. Clontarf. A seemingly innocuous north Dublin suburb where the rich coexist in apparent peace with the even richer. And yet' – my voice here rose with the still raw emotion – 'Brian Boru, High King of All Ireland, was savagely murdered there as he lay relaxing in his tent. Admittedly this happened a long time ago – 1014 to be precise – but it still has the power to shock.'

I whittled a marrow into the shape of a medieval axe – a symptom, perhaps, of my inner turmoil – and wiped away a tear or two of rage.

'Your point?' snapped my solitary customer.

'My point,' I said, gently and not without love, 'is that wounds heal slowly. So put the gun down. Have a tossed salad on the house.' I dropped my voice to a truth and reconciliation whisper. 'Let it go.'

***

'But he didn't let it go, Een. Did he?'

(QUIET) 'No.'

'It might have been better if he had. Not for us to say it was a bit on the long side, but two Brazilian rain forests for the first print run?'

'Anyway, "Sloot" is a more manageable size. Well done, by the way. It's a veritable hoot.'

'You won't have read it yourself, of course, being as what you wrote it. (SIGH) *Poor old Willie Shakespeare, dough. He died some years later. And you know something? He's never been the same since.'*

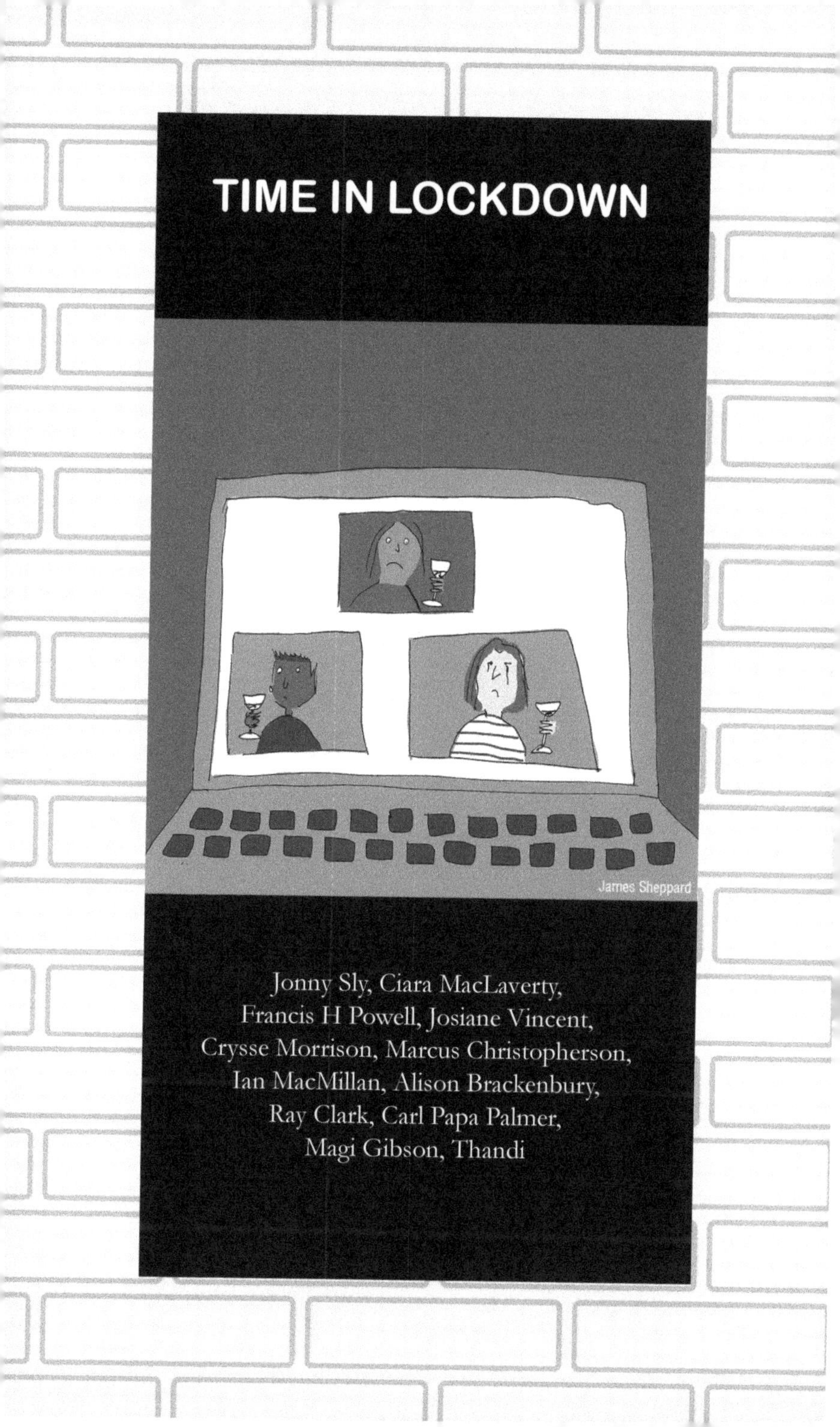
TIME IN LOCKDOWN
James Sheppard
Jonny Sly, Ciara MacLaverty,
Francis H Powell, Josiane Vincent,
Crysse Morrison, Marcus Christopherson,
Ian MacMillan, Alison Brackenbury,
Ray Clark, Carl Papa Palmer,
Magi Gibson, Thandi

Dawn Chorus

Jonny Sly

the birds are tweeting
not for me or for you
the dawn is bleating
grey sky drifting to blue
the trees are still bones
the crows are already getting stoned
my tongue is turning to glue
spring is springing and
somewhere the young
lambs are waiting
for the night of the long
knives and easter confined
inside ovens
eyes like buttons
coming undone
a face like trousers
falling round ankles
good job nobody can see
the arse insomnia makes of me
(until you read my poetry)

Day 52

Ciara MacLaverty

At first, it sounded exciting.
Lockdown: the title of a cult film
or the chorus of a rap anthem.
Lockdown! Shockdown!
We ain't driving round town!

Stay home. Stay sane. Next day, do it again.
Our garden pond is the size of a double bed,
with water like a school paint pot
near the end of Double Art.
Below the weeds, a pair of goldfish glow,
orange sweets from *Quality Street.*

I throw confetti flakes,
seaweed scent on fingertips
and wait for the thin *plip*
of mouths on surface,
a mermaid flick of tails, their finest minute.
The city air was never fresher, more astringent.

The kids are starting up the Xbox.
Five scruffy footballs lie chewed in our own goal.
It's Thursday, isn't it?
A squirrel, drenched by sunlight, stops and starts,
his tail a *back-to-front* question mark.

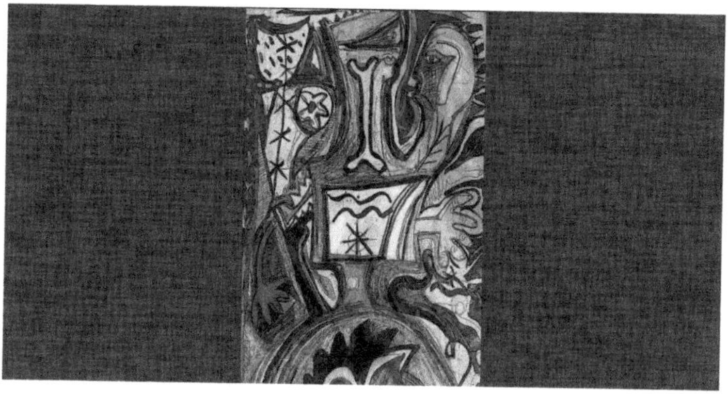

Lockdown

Francis H Powell & Jonny Sly

Are you walking on sunshine,
or leaping cloud to cloud
with repetitive ease
thoughts floating in the breeze
the world shoved to one side
opera ringing in your mind
dancing in the empty streets
roses showering at your feet?

Or are you fighting with the kids
as they kick and punch your inner peace
bouncing off the walls
as their energy overflows
another day of lockdown goes
day twenty four twenty five
another day less alive?

I'm hunched up like a stowaway
holed up in the hold
rocking on my sit bones
teeth and knees clenching
my stomach wrenching
as the ship heaves up and down
blind to its direction
oblivious to its inclinations
I've given up cutting notches on the beam
forgotten what they mean
losing count loses the mind
even numbers feel confined

Are your hours long and lumpish
or are they plump with good intentions
thinking of the pensioner
who cannot shop
been forced to cut herself off
from the company of kith and kin
nobody coming in
nobody to hear her sighing?

Maybe it's all trippy or trying
taxing or strangely satisfying
as you wrestle with its every manifestation
locked down in irresistible infection fascination
trying to make sense of the signification
of the hydra-headed bestiary
that assails you in this dark dream
which now seems all too real?

Have you battened down the hatches
diving in your inner submarine

on a voyage of self-discovery
twenty thousand leagues under the me?
Or are you the king of your desert island
riding the seahorses, surfing the scallops
blowing on a conch
that clarion call
that summons the sirens who sing you to sleep
if only you knew where to fall?

Or have you set adrift on a raft to
see where the storm tides cast you
glass seas
and sunsets
the essence of solace
a shooting star an albatross
flying fish
a dolphin's click
a humpback whale
surging into sight shooting water skywards
a rousing snort
the flick of the tail fin then back in
and down
down
down
down
as if it never was there
as if you were never here
but lost on the horizon of your dreams
anything is possible right now
even you
sometimes?

Are you having a house party in your head
the smiling guests toasting your very good health

leading them on a merry dance
arms and legs akimbo
your dear friendships in limbo
(better turn the music down
the neighbours might complain
think your lockdown busting
too scared you've gone insane
already deafened by the sound of their own pain
nerves sucked away down their own brain drain)
glasses chink amid chattering and mirth
can I offer you nuts
oh I am sorry love
clean forgot
about your allergy
and the problem of the calories
well try my humus dip
a recipe tip
I picked up
from the Middle East
Orient Express delivery
tried and tested over the centuries
a mystery of history
or perhaps you'd like a cup of tea
come on get up get happy
the party must go on
no bounds no borders
keep on keeping on
keep it up so it goes on too long
is that wrong?

Or you could be hooked to your computer?
connecting and disseminating
distance learning

or video demonstrating
telling strangers how to be stranger still
killing the time they're dying to kill
a ping from an old friend
who surges into mind
what a fine time you had back when
and you regret the years lost and then
news of a mother giving birth
it's her fourth another girl
one more blond-haired highlight
in a flourishing family
of golden-locked delights
see that Father's smile
a joy to behold
holding the baby
haloed in gold
or friends' children
penned up in the garden
playing with tin cans and pots and pans
or whatever they can get their hands on
as spring kicks in
its shoots shooting
through the ceiling
into an empty limpid sky
as blue as you
and your question why?

Life reels on
like some drunk sailor
lurching down the street
his heart fractured
his song dismembered
his feet

tangled in his memories
laughing and sobbing
as he stumbles into walls
and he won't sleep
he'll keep us up
pining for the open sea
until he sups some kind of release
however slowly
but he knows truly
how every teaspoon
of relief
on his lips
will taste oh so sweet

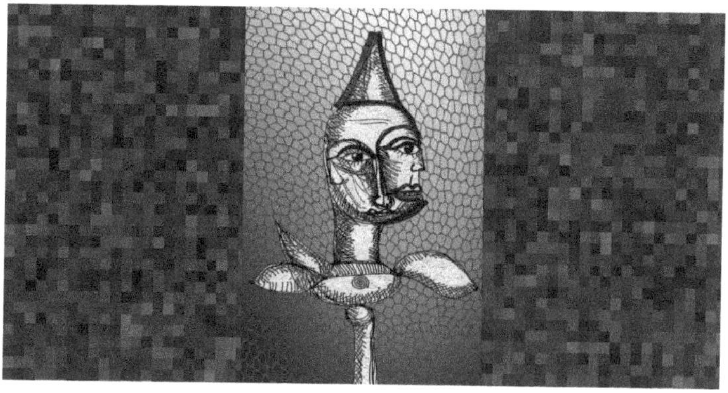

Time Passing

Jonny Sly

Time? oh aye,
indeed
it's passing
doing that a lot these days is Time
at the door comes knocking
and says how do? just asking
come in for a cuppa I reply
but Time just sighs
sorry can't, just passing by
all right, see you round some time
ha funny that
some Time
that's a bit of you, that is
you're everywhere
here and there
high time downtime
half-time full-time
lunchtime bedtime

lost time war time
good time bad time
big time small time
that's why you think you're so great
but really you're inadequate
not got enough You
for everyone
so you never have a mo
for a biscuit and banter
always just passing
always just asking
how do?
rushing on
and then you're gone
never enough of you
to pass the time of day
idle the afternoon away
go, be off you
you and me, we're through
and by that point I've got quite miffed
and I've gone and turned the kettle off
getting none of my tea, that one, just plain rude
I mutter to myself
tidying the teabags back on the shelf
(anyway Time likes its brew cold and stewed)
in hindsight I guess Time's not being all that gruff
gets invitations enough
to stop off for tea and stuff
so if Time keeps passing
and never popping in
and never stopping by
it's cos Time's just social distancing
that's the thing

like me and you
it's the only thing Time can do
in case, we catch that contagion that is new
I mean, imagine catching crazy bat flu thing
from Time

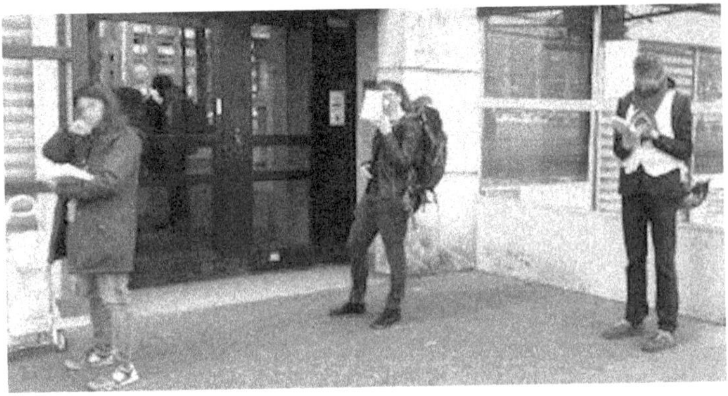

Time Sparing

Josiane Vincent

Time for reading
Time for waiting
Time for thinking
Time for hoping
The clock of time is ticking away
As mirrored beyond a shop window
Secretive "ombres chinoises"
Seem to be conspiring in
A scenery of buildings and trees reflected
And who are these people
Standing on the open air stage
Of an haphazard theatre?
Let me guess!
They are actors in their own living role
In an improbable play
Anonymous characters
voiceless
No script

No plot
They are not performing
Not even posing
Perhaps just rehearsing
Open books in hands
Engrossed
As off stage
A photographer that happened
To be passing by
off handedly
snapped this triad
A scene out of the ordinary
A souvenir of Paris
On an endless day of confinement

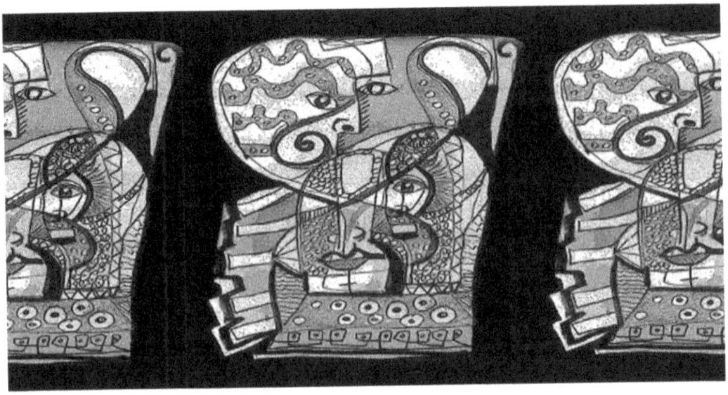

Where Did the Week Go

Jonny Sly

In a month of Sundays
I never mused I'd mourn a Monday
Tomorrow never comes
Let alone a Tuesday
Wednesday's is now When's-the-day?
Full of wheres, whos and whats?
And Thursday's an absurd day
Observed only by covidiots
Don't thank God it's never Friday
Is not something I thought I'd say
And I cannot leave early
Because tomorrow won't be Saturday
Saturday will never come
Saturday won't be live
Saturday's another sorry day
Just as messed as the other five

Like a mask to a face
to Sunday
stuck we are forever
anxious for days
and living the never

Ten weeks in

Crysse Morrison

Walking in sunshine
Ashamed of my happiness
So many so sad

This plague has taught me
more than I wanted to know
about some friendships

This plague has assured
strength of one relationship
despite all my doubts

Still

Marcus Christopherson

Time has stood still,
Yet faster than ever.
Heavier than steel,
Light as a feather.

Invisible enemy,
Plain to see,
Who's to blame?
Not, I or me.

Closer than knit,
Harder to sever,
Forever alone,
Always together.

Stronger as one,
Even stronger apart,
We celebrate life,
But mourn from a far.

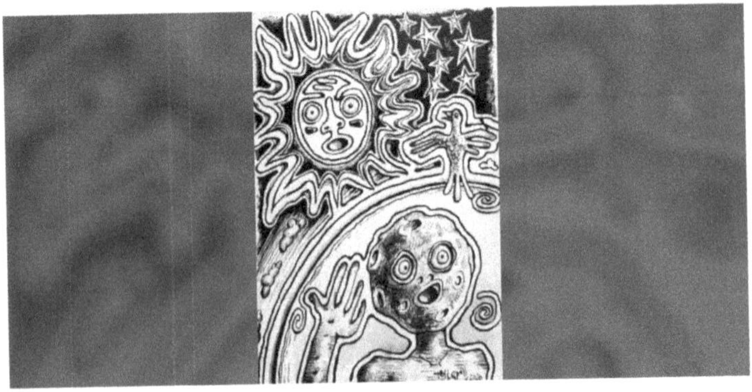

Sun and Moon

Ian MacMillan

Sun and moon
In the same sky
Isolated, distancing

In time zones
Neither would recognise.
One sweating, one not.

Me and you
On the same lawn
Clipping, gazing

In time zones
Cracked and shrunk, the ones
2020 cooked for us

Offered
As serving suggestions.
That bird seems to fly

Between the sun
And the moon,
in no time at all.

Sunday on the coach

Alison Brackenbury

It is June. Tall grasses nod. On the back seat
the last baby has hiccupped into sleep.
No one swears, nobody phones. The south wind whistles
white motorways of cow parsley and thistles.
A helicopter hangs, but does not strafe.
This afternoon the innocent are safe.

Ranger Man

Ray Clark

'What is a man profited, if he shall gain the whole world, and lose his own soul?'
[The Bible – King James Version]

Cassandra pulled into a vacant space and shut off the engine. Scattered around were perhaps another dozen vehicles at the most, one of which was a brand new, white Ford Ranger. The owner was lowering the tailgate.

Leaving the car she pressed the fob to lock it, rubbing her hands across her face, struggling to believe how tired she was: reflecting on a twenty-four-hour shift from hell at the hospital, mostly without a break because they simply didn't have the staff to cope with the deluge of patients, not to mention adequate PPE.

Shopping was the last thing on her mind, especially if the rumours were true. Empty shelves due to panic buying; increased prices due to profiteering: people arguing, almost fighting over what was left. The list was endless.

She popped a pound coin into the trolley, dragged it out of the line and headed in through the glass doors.

"I wouldn't bother if I was you, love," said the old dear with the blue rinse, on her way out. "Bugger all on the shelves … well nothing anybody wants. I think it's disgraceful."

Cassandra's stomach swelled. Maybe the stories had been true. Once inside the entrance she saw for herself. Most of the aisles were deserted, with only a handful of shoppers, wandering aimlessly, glancing vacantly.

The baskets at the front of the store containing the fresh bread and pastries were all empty. Cass found that disappointing, not for herself but for her seven-year-old daughter, Sophie, who loved the Portuguese custard tarts.

As she pushed the trolley further forward the story was the same. No bread, breadcakes, eggs or any other staples.

Surely to God it wasn't happening.

All she needed was enough food for the two of them tonight, to 0return home for a nice hot shower, sort out the meal, a glass of wine, and spend time with Sophie.

She headed further into the meat and fresh veg section. Two women argued over a steak, pulling the package back and forth. If they continued it wouldn't be worth having anyway. An elderly gent watched on anxiously.

"I've told you, it's mine," said the redhead.

"It isn't, it's his," replied the blonde, pointing to the elderly gent. "You pulled it out of his hand."

"I have a family to feed."

"And he has a disabled wife."

"And I have three sons, all still working, supporting the economy. Keeping the likes of his wife, I shouldn't wonder."

Everyone was horrified by that statement.

"Ladies," said the elderly gent, "there really is no need for this."

"There you are," said the redhead, "he's letting me have it."

"I'm sure that's not what he meant," replied the blonde.

"I don't care what he meant."

Cass noticed that the redhead actually had *three* packets of steak in total – two were already in the basket, and the last ones as far as she could see. "They're mine," she pointed a warning finger, "and neither you, nor him, nor anyone else in this place is gonna take them from me."

The elderly gent sighed and turned his trolley round as the redhead stormed off. The blonde shrugged her shoulders and said sorry to him, but it wasn't her fault. What she *did* do was give him her only piece of meat.

Cass apologised to him and it hadn't even involved her.

Further into the store it was the same story. The shelves with all the tinned goods were empty: no pasta either. The kitchen and toilet rolls had gone, as if the place had been looted.

Cass felt like lead inside. How was she going to explain to her daughter? She suspected the rest of the shops would be no better.

In the end, all she managed was some washing powder and a packet of out-of-date ham on the cheap shelf. Further sorrowful expressions from the checkout staff only added to her despair.

With her one carrier bag she strolled out of the supermarket with a heavy heart, wondering how she was going to concoct a satisfactory meal for either of them.

In the car park, a very heated discussion with the driver of the new Ford Ranger and a couple of other shoppers – each with near empty trolleys – was underway.

As she strolled toward them she noticed, on the back of his pick up, that he had a pack of twenty-four toilet rolls, which he was selling for a pound each.

"Arsehole," shouted a teenager, filming it, "you ought to be ashamed of yourself."

"Look, do you want one, or don't you?" asked Ranger man.

"Not at your bloody prices we don't," said a middle-aged lady.

The elderly gent with a disabled wife thought differently. He bought two, said he needed them whatever the cost.

"What's he doing?" Cass asked another middle-aged man.

"He's just bought the last packet in there, love," he replied, pointing to the supermarket. She noticed what she thought was the manager at the entrance, watching the development.

"What?" said Cass, "and now he's selling them for a pound each?"

"Aye."

She saw red. A nurse she may be, and trained to save lives,

but right now she felt like taking one. Other items on his vehicle included ready meals priced up at five pounds each, and a number of cuts of meat, most with yellow labels on, tagged up as much as twenty pounds each.

"People like you disgust me," said Cass.

"I have a family to feed, love. Now do you want something, or don't you?"

"And a brand new Ranger to run," added Cass. "I'm a nurse, I've just worked a twenty four hour shift in the hospital without a break. All I came here for was some food to feed my daughter, and a few personal items and there's nothing left on the shelves."

"My heart bleeds for you, love. But don't worry, I've got plenty on the back of here."

"Nobody is buying anything from you," said the man who had been standing at the entrance to the supermarket. His name badge informed them he was the manager. "Now take your stuff and get out of here before I call the police." He had his phone in his hand.

"I've got nothing to feed my daughter with tonight," shouted Cass. "You should be ashamed of yourself, profiteering in such trying times."

"Like I said, love, there's plenty on here," shouted Ranger man, smiling.

"It's alright, girl," said one of the female shoppers. She reached into her basket and pulled out a lasagne. "It's not much but I'm not as desperate as you sound. Does your daughter like lasagne?"

"Here, love," said another, passing over a loaf of wholemeal bread.

Another said, "I've got some beans here, nurse."

A lady offered half a dozen eggs.

Cass broke down in floods of tears at the generosity. "I can't," she said, "I really shouldn't. What are *you* going to do?"

"Don't worry about us, love," said the elderly gent with the disabled wife. "Some of us fought in the war, we know what it's like to have nothing, and we know the value of friendship, and sharing." He glanced at Ranger man. "If I was twenty years younger…"

"You'd what, old man? Get yourself home, it's past your bedtime."

The old man lifted his walking cane.

"If you're still here in five minutes," shouted the supermarket manager, "I'm calling the police."

Ranger man grunted and closed the tailgate.

"You'll get your comeuppance, son, don't you worry," shouted one of the shoppers, as he stalked away.

"Yes," shouted another, "what goes around comes around."

"What does that even mean?" replied Ranger man, jumping in his vehicle.

A discussion continued for another five minutes, in which Cass could not thank the people enough.

Later in the evening she cried herself to sleep. She'd made sure Sophie had eaten, who'd asked her mother why she wasn't eating.

Cass said she'd had something in the hospital canteen and all she wanted was a shower. After Sophie had gone to bed, she'd made a cup of tea with beans on toast. It was heaven.

***

Three days later, she was back on shift, having been put in charge of the Covid ward. It was an awful sight, full to the brim with people who had breathing difficulties and who would be lucky to survive the night.

She studied the report of the first she came to. His name was Stephen James Walker. He'd been admitted that morning with mild symptoms, which had become full blown by mid afternoon. A ventilator now helped him.

She replaced his chart and went over to introduce herself, to tell him that she would be doing everything in her power to make sure he was as comfortable as she could make him.

Cass received a shock when she saw the man staring back at her. He couldn't speak, but he implored her with his eyes to help him.

Professional to the last she said that if there was anything he wanted he only had to ring the bell.

As she turned, she couldn't help but wonder if Ranger man had managed to sell everything on his vehicle that night, and what he'd spent the profit on.

Whatever it was, it was of no use to him now.

In Praise of Stay-At-Home

Carl Papa Palmer

Our days used to begin in a frantic rush
led by Mom herding everyone to wake up,
wash up, eat up and hurry up out the door.

Everyone except me, I never got to go.
My days were spent alone in the house
waiting for everyone to come back home.

I'd make my rounds, look under beds,
check the bathrooms and kitchen then
nap on the couch for the rest of my day.

I live with Mom, Dad, Sissy and Bubba
on a street full of families and their pets.
Our pet is me, a boxer. I answer to Bob.

I don't know why or what happened, but
everybody stayed home one day, all day
and every day since. I am one lucky dog!

I get more walks, more bow wows with my
buddies and their masked masters, though
not close enough for our usual social sniff.
More snacks, more playing, more petting,
more snuggling, best is not being alone,
but I do miss my long naps on the couch.

April 2020

Magi Gibson

A child's voice bounces through the open window
of the lockdown house next door. In our garden
tulips flounce scarlet hussy petticoats, daffodils
bounce out golden notes, a chaffinch chirrucks
in a willow tree, catkin buds burst yellow,
fat and merry, cherry trees blush pink as candy-floss.
No constant traffic roar nearby. No white contrails
of planes criss-cross the sky. A perfect spring!
But for the distant sound of siren wails
that drift from time to time, invisible ribbons
in the dangerous air. They catch us unaware,
bind round our throats, constrain us as we isolate
and wait, uncertain what each day will bring
in this exuberant, this strangely fearful spring.

Hiber-Nation

Thandi

Forced into hibernation, like a bear in winter
In my room with Netflix on constant rotation
Cozied up with my snacks instead of a pint of bitter
Eating my way to obesity, the only city that is inviting

London city is temporarily shut
I can't really do much
Except eat warm waffles and ice-cream
And escape inside my laptop screen

With no living room for socialising
I distracted myself from the pain of isolation
I binge watched till I overdosed
Choking on the realisation that human interaction
matters most.

LONELINESS AND EMPTINESS

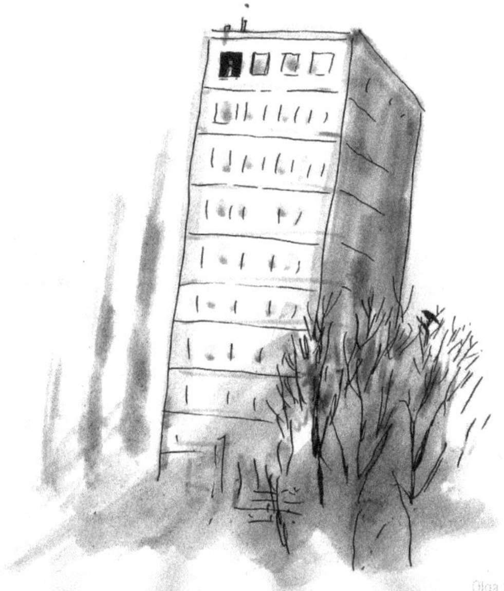

Olga Solabarrieta

Julie C. Round, Josiane Vincent, Fizzy Twizler, Moique Tell, Crystal Turner-Brightman, Monica Shah, Francis H Powell, Joyce West, Giselle Marks, Connie Howell, Johnnie Dalton, Carmina Masoliver, Jane Lovell, Laura Zuwa Ukpokolo, Karl Nova, Aoife Mannix, Seadeta Osmani, Andy J. Tyler

Covid 19

Julie C. Round

While danger lurks outside the home
We must remain inside, alone.
I've books to read, letters to write
Meals to prepare, TV at night-
Surely that will be quite enough
To stop this purdah being tough?

But deep into the isolation
There came a very strange sensation.
I wondered what would happen if
I died, and while I was a stiff
Others would rummage through my litter
And rage and sigh and become bitter
At all the stuff I'd left behind
Too much, I'm sure, for them to find
The gems of writing I had got,
Instead, they'd chuck the bloomin' lot.

So, miserably, I set to sort
The paper mountain that I ought
To have destroyed months, years, before
Then made a pile upon the floor.
I ripped and shredded sheets and bills
And found some empty bags to fill
And saved them to add to the bin.
A task I knew I could not win-

At first I read, then tore and ripped
But then my good intentions slipped
Photos of holidays long gone
With maps and brochures, it felt wrong
To destroy all that history
Memories meant so much to me.
So while some papers are destroyed
Some still remain to make annoyed
The people who come after me-
Next week I'll still a hoarder be!

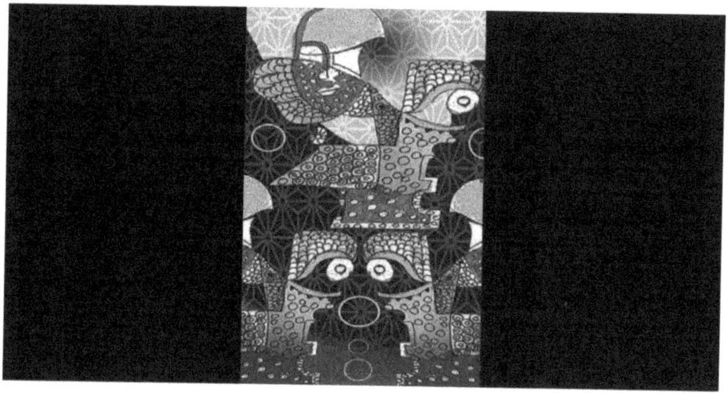

Day Dream

Josiane Vincent

The streets are empty
I am walking in the mist
Muffled voices
throbbing in my ears
Ghastly figures
Brushing past me
What is this strange voice
Calling me from deep down?
This is but a dream

I am floating over the oceans
Surrounded by seagulls
A seagull myself
I'm looking down
Below
A strange shadow
wading through the waves
is beckoning at me

When I fly down closer
I can see that it is
But my reflection in the waters

The beach is quiet
For a sunny afternoon
Not a soul
For miles around
Except for a dog
On an errand
Total confinement is the rule

I am pushing open a hidden door
It reveals a secret path
I am wrapped in stillness
Over there I can glimpse
Flimsy shadows
With a mask over
Their mouth and nose
They are gliding on the Acheron
It is but my imagination

A gentle wind is blowing
Through my hair
Leaves are swivelling down
They are but unwritten pages
I pick one up
A blank page
To tell unheard stories
A blank page
To record the confinement
A blank page
To write a new world
But it is yet to be invented.

The Lonely

Fizzy Twizler

Pleas for help
Across all borders
And the seven seas
Isolation everywhere
Separated confused lonely

Empty restaurants
Empty playgrounds
Children elderly dazed lonely

No one hears
No time to care
The end maybe very near
But time never said
Go ahead be lonely

How about together
We face this monster
Stay at home but
Don't forget the lonely

2020 plague we have the technology
There's no need to feel lonely.

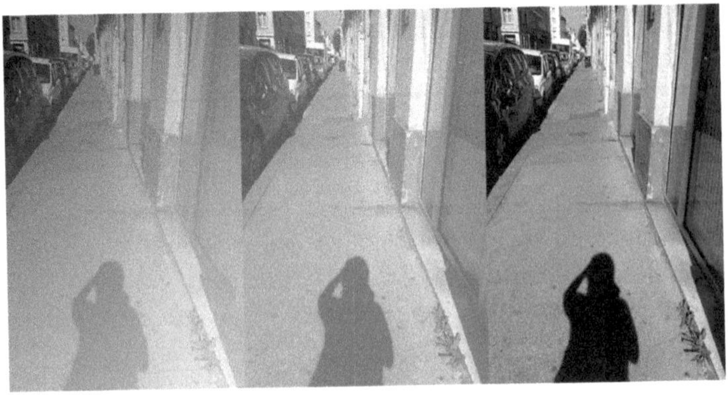

Isolation

Monique Tell

I didn't move. Stayed standing at the closed kitchen window for most of the morning, peering into the motionless sky, gazing at its sickening blue, trying to forget the explosion of spring on the hill before me and its flourishing trees doomed to drought. Even the rain has come to a standstill.

I turn to watch the almost deserted square, the comings and goings of now familiar forms, the indolence of a woman in a mask, pushing a stroller bearing a baby in a mask, dozing, the manic elation of two children (both masked) on their tiny shiny bikes, the helmet-headed patrol who steps out then steps back into their truck as white as their masks, the docile queue at the cornershop, sensibly tidy, each at the regulation 1 meter, 1 meter, 1 meter distance behind the orange stripes stuck to the ground: The queue for the bakery, spans to the corner of the square, snakes around the broad dumb brasserie, and disappears off into the boulevard.

In a shambles, the impertinent sparrows have come back to inhabit the neighborhood, perched in the trees, tucked in the holes of the stone walls and nestled beneath the red tiles of the gables. From six in the morning I can already hear them chirping their joie de vivre above the city. They hop across the dry pink baked earth of the square. In search of something? What might they hope to find? Stunned by the sudden abundance of feathers, a cat scatters in the nick of time from beneath the wheels of a slaloming scooter, out of control. I want him here. I want him to live with me. How do you call to a cat?

My neighbor across the hall, my "door mat" neighbour, I call her, knocks softly at the door, a sign she has hung a bag on the handle. Probably the old magazines she reads from which I glean some outdated news. What does it matter playing catch-up? Surely any news dates from the moment it is said? At least that is how it feels, so used are we to hindsight.

I put the potatoes to boil and I hear the water gently lapping around them. Done as many as I can, so as not to worry about cooking. A boiled potato, a bowl of crudités, a wedge of cheese. Got enough in to hold out for a while.

I think of the fragrance of fig trees in the summer South, the joys of plucking fruit from the tree, biting into the sweet, scented, purple flesh, I think of cherries and grapes, their color, their flavor, their sensuality. I think of everything I love and I miss it like I may never taste it again. My mouth is watering, my eyes are weeping.

The song of the telephone and cell phone never ceasing. News from afar, how life is now clean, hygienic, economical. We've all stopped spending and expending ourselves. Instead we stand at windows, thinking, our arms hanging, empty.

When will we savour the endless rowdy aperitifs, devour the prodigal barbecues, feel the family's warm embrace, see sweethearts smooching, "I want to get smashed on Mort Subite, get wasted by a shot in the dark of eau de vie, I want to feel you, your arms and your lips, like burning Claquesin intoxicating my skin!"

Wishbone

Dennis Copelan

After eighty-three days in lockdown, things had gotten tense. It was hard enough for three twenty-year old, unemployed college students to live in a two-bedroom apartment, but add in a slobbering dog loudly chewing on a chew bone, and tempers wore thin.

"Who gave Coco another chew bone?" I hollered, irritated by the slurping, grinding, and licking.

"I did," said Monique, leaning out from the kitchen wearing a black butcher's apron that matched the color of her hair. "She loves them."

I pursed my lips. "You know she's on a gluten-free diet? It upsets her digestive system."

Monique feigned a frown. "But she looked so sad."

Shaking my head, I put my Kindle on the couch, and pried the slimy dog treat away from Coco. The poodle's sad eyes tried to guilt me, but I wouldn't let her. I wiped my hands on my baggy grey sweats.

Fletcher, looking like he'd just awakened, shaggy and unshaved, wandered in from his bedroom, wearing no shirt. As he ambled in the cuffs of his ratty pajama bottoms dragged across the carpeted floor. "Hey," he said. "Wha's for lunch?"

Monique smiled, "Macaroni and cheese."

"Again?" I complained.

"Yeah, no pizza?" yawned Fletcher.

The grin faded from Monique's face. "Listen, I'm tired of cooking for you guys. If you want something different, maybe you should put on masks, get out of the apartment and go grocery shopping." She glared at me. "Right, Chloe?"

Before I could answer there were two loud bangs on the apartment door that startled us all. Coco barked.

"What the hell?" I blurted.

Fletcher, clearly worried, wrinkled his brow. "Did we pay the rent?"

"Go see who it is," said Monique.

I glanced at both of them and realized neither one would check. Running my hand through my uncombed blond hair, I walked over to the peephole and looked. Coco followed me. She sniffed the door.

"Is it pizza?"

"It's a packing envelope," I said, squinting. "Did anyone order anything?"

Fletcher plopped on the couch. "With what money?"

Monique shrugged. "Not me."

I retrieved my gloves and bleach spray.

After disinfecting the mysterious envelope, I brought it inside, holding the rectangle away from me with my index finger and thumb.

The three of us grabbed seats around the kitchen table, eyeing the unmarked envelope like the thing bore an array of Egyptian hieroglyphics.

Coco lay near our feet, appearing as sad as ever.

"Who would send a plain envelope?" I asked.

Fletcher brightened. "Maybe it's drugs?" After I gave him a hard look, he lowered his gaze. "Just sayin'," he muttered.

Monique lifted the thin manila envelope and shook it. "It feels like a letter."

I snitched it from her hands, ripped it open and pulled out the note. Adjusting my glasses, I read the correspondence.

Monique seemed intrigued. "Who's it from?" she asked.

"Just somebody's idea of a stupid joke. From the Wish Foundation."

Fletcher leaned back. "What's it say, Chloe?"

"It says we were picked randomly. We're entitled to one wish for anything we want. No request denied." I flipped the letter onto the table. "What a bunch of crap!"

Fletcher snatched it up. "Lemme see that. Maybe it's real."

Monique read the offer over Fletcher's shoulder. "What if it's true?" she reflected.

I rolled my eyes. "You've gotta be kidding."

"I think it's legit," said Fletcher.

"How would you know?"

"Hey, I know things," he said in all seriousness.

"Like what?"

"Like secret ancient societies. The Illuminati. The Knights of the Golden Circle. The Order of the Skull and Bones. The Freemasons. The Merry Marvel Marching Society."

"The Merry Marvel Marching Society? Who are they?" I asked.

"I don't know. I saw an ad for it in an old Spider-Man comic book." Fletcher stared past a wall. "It's always been a mystery to me."

"You're an idiot."

"No, wait," said Monique. "What if Fletcher's right? Supposing some secret society randomly picked us. What would you do with a wish?"

"Magic isn't real," I exclaimed.

"Au contraire," opined Fletcher. "What if it's metaphysical science?"

"What does that even mean?"

"It means, let's make a wish," said Monique.

Coco peered up at me. She put her paw on my thigh and whimpered.

"No, Coco. You can't have your chew treat back."

The dog slid to the floor and sighed.

"Since there's three of us, why don't we each say what we want," suggested Monique.

"You can't do that." said Fletcher. "The moment one of us wishes for something, we've used it up. We have to be methodical."

"Okay then, we'll just have to agree on it," she said. "What would you want, Fletcher?"

"Pizza."

I lashed out. "That's what you'd wish for? The greatest power in the world, and you'd want to fill your stomach with a pizza? What about helping your fellow man? Like asking for peace or curing Covid or cancer?

"Or feeding the hungry?" Monique added.

Fletcher flopped his head forward, desperation in his voice. "But I'm hungry."

His response made me sneer. "This is useless."

"What a minute," said Monique, her eyes widening. "What if we made our wish like one long run-on sentence? Why, we could ask for anything."

"No, you couldn't, it's still one wish," I argued.

Fletcher raised his head. "She's right. They didn't send anyone here to verify."

"How do you know?"

"Because there's no genie. You need a lamp for a genie. All we got was a lousy letter."

"Do you hear yourself?" I said. "I can't believe we're even having this discussion."

Monique handed out some paper and pens. "We should write down all the things we want. When we're ready, Chloe will say, 'I wish' and read everything on our lists—real fast—so the Foundation will think it's one request."

"Why me?" I protested. "Why not him? I don't even believe in this."

"Because they'd take you seriously." She nodded to Fletcher. "Just look at him."

Fletcher frantically wrote his list. "How do you spell Toblerone?"

Resigned, I took pen to paper and jotted down my own list. When I finished, I asked, "Ready?"

Monique and Fletcher handed me their pages.

"Okay," I said. I spread the sheets on the table.

"Don't forget to read really fast," said Monique.

Coco barked twice.

"Quiet Coco!" I took a deep breath. "I wish…"

And then we heard a loud crunch and gnawing under the table.

I stopped. "What's that noise?"

Coco dragged out a large all-natural chew bone twice her size. She lay on the ground and munched away.

"Who gave her that bone?" I accused.

"I didn't," said Monique.

"Me neither," said Fletcher.

We all looked at Coco and then at the Wish Foundation letter on the table.

My face fell slack. "Oh. Coco…."

Fletcher picked up the letter and tore it in half. He slumped back in his chair.

I sighed.

"Who wants macaroni and cheese?" asked Monique.

Inside Isolation

Crystal Turner-Brightman

Isolation is so hard when you feel cold and alone
Standing looking round thinking home isn't home
You're with the people you love but there's more you need to see
Every day, every second, becomes an eternity
You look out the window but there's nowhere to go
The world that was, isn't there to show
I know this poem is sad but what else can I do
I can't pretend to be happy, when I'm feeling so blue
I know it won't be forever, but right now it is
When there's people I want to hold and people I miss
Loved ones who are gone I won't see again
It makes me want to grab the here ones even closer and then
I want to wrap them in love and protect them from harm
But I know that I can't, so instead I sit calm
I hold close who I can and reach out to the others
In times like these, you must look out for one another.

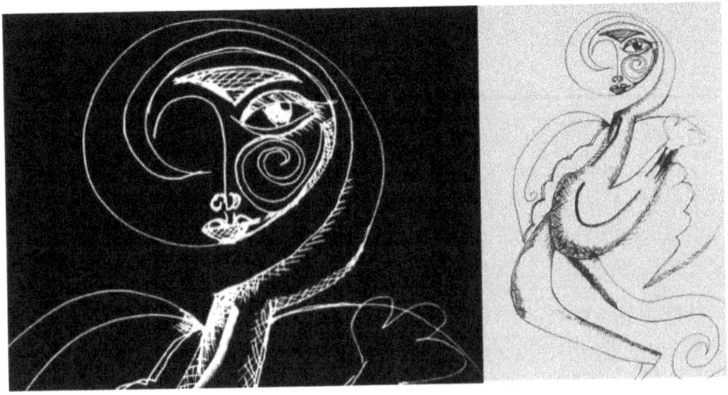

There Was an Old Woman

Monica Shah

She was 81 when her wrinkled hands began to shake
while drinking her tea. Her arms, once slender
and adorned in gold bangles were freckled in sunspots.

Her history told in the road map of swollen veins
marking her legs, her slack skin speckled and sallow,
her face a dusty mask of papery folds, cobweb-soft.

A mole above her lip sprouted 2 wiry hairs. She cried
out for her daughters "Aria, please come" and
"Maggie, where are you?" Hours later perhaps someone

stopped by. She called out "my son, my son"
over and over and sometimes he would say something
about seeing her tomorrow. Eventually no one answered

when she called and no one held her hand anymore.
Soon her hands stopped shaking and her voice went silent.
Then there were no more tomorrows at all.

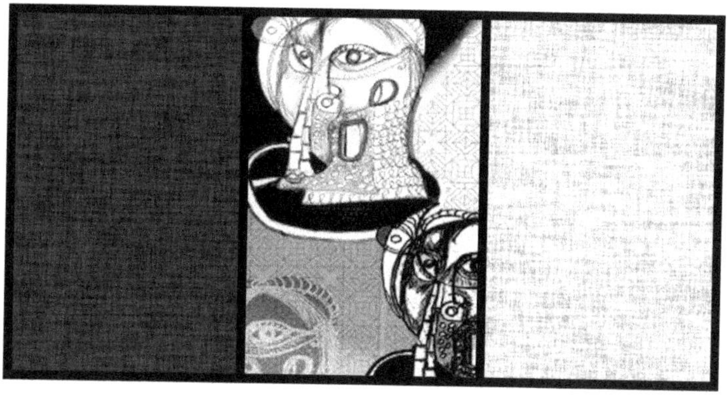

Unity

Francis H Powell

Empty trains going nowhere
Churches where the choirs don't sing
A lonely Gothic opera
A party with no people, the sound of silence
The doorbell never rings
Open roads that lead to oblivion
Find a way, yes find a way
Windows that look out to emptiness
doors that lead to a nothingness void
A restaurant open to nobody
The cooks food left to rot and fester
Queens with meaningless speeches
with crowns upon their heads
banishing jesters from their sacred palaces
Dust gathering in schools and parks
Dreamers walking round in hope
Lovers capturing moments together
Heroes setting about their work

caring for those in need
Gods looking down on human chaos
Birds building nests
joggers turning in circles
dogs pulling their owners
in all kinds of directions.

Aged souls wondering what is happening
How can this be?
Recriminations, pointed fingers
can we all do better?
Where's the hope, where is the way out?
Business men fussing and fretting
as their money drains away
As one day turns into another
The news tells us a new story
Planes grounded
The homeless hunting for a haven
The afflicted turning thoughts in their minds
The waves still crashing on empty shores
Wanderers wandering for ever
welcome to the lost tribes of nirvana my dear
beggars looking for scraps of food
children bored, nothing to do
mindless television, time moves slowly
Pick up the pieces from all the remains
and find your inner soul
Come on mankind pull yourself together.

Waiting for Ted

Joyce West

She sits in the window looking,
For what I know not,
But every day the same
I pass by, a quick look,
Then avert my eyes.
I ask a neighbour who she is
She shrugs her shoulders
And says she doesn't know
I almost forget as I pass by
That's she's sitting there
In a high back chair
With her silver hair
Looking through me
Or is it beyond until one day
She's not there, gone.

That evening I worry
After all she's always there.
So I knock on the door
And wait and wait
I knock again and listen
A faint call, a voice,
So I dial for the police
Thinking she's had a fall.
They go round the back
Over the wall
And yes I was right
She's had a bad fall.
She's semi-conscious

But she holds my hand tight
So I go with her to hospital.
We're there all night.
They send her home in a cab
With me still by her side.
I have her keys.

So we go into the kitchen
I make the tea and look around.
She's gone back
To her chair in the window.
I kneel take her hand
And ask who is it you wait for.
She smiles and says my Ted
Not yet but soon he'll be here,
I've waited ten years.
I ask where he's been
She smiles, says don't be silly
He's dead but he always said
He'd come back for me
So I must be ready
And look my best
So you go home
While I wait for him.

Self-Isolation

Giselle Marks

Three score and five years with children flown
Isolation the norm no woman is an island sole
Friends are wanted and friends die
Younger yet their time has come and
I must wish them sad farewell.
Rebuild a life and make new friends
Covid comes I must imprison myself from risk.

Not a cell – more house arrest
Only leaving for sustenance
Little hope of quick relief
No appeal for innocence
No parole for good behaviour
No hugs, no kisses, no smiles
From those I pass in hope
That I am far enough away.

My island home is not worst hit
But anyone could be a carrier
Friends, neighbours we must shun
Until the virus goes or a cure is found.
Strange existence unsocial
Linked only by electronic means.

Some governments have done well
To lessen the number who fall sick
Some nations found it harder to abide
The poor and rich countries suffer more

Nations unprepared for such infection
Suffering physical and financial
As masses fear human contact
And hide away in their dwellings.

My small town is quiet, few cars pass
A few dog walkers walk on by
But do not stop to talk or smile
Keeping a distance from anyone out
I shop and race back home
Alone once more I am on my own.

Covid 19 Isolation

Connie Howell

I may be in isolation but I am not alone
You are out there also
One heart amongst many

It may have taken a virus to unite us
To bring creativity to the fore
New ideas and opportunities, creation at its best

Many people are caught in a web of fear
Insane shopping, pushing, shoving
Scarcity on their minds

Panic of "not enough" and "what ifs"
Some becoming their worst selves
Others finding their best, their inner kindness

Same virus, different response

Nature has given us the chance to reflect
To dig deep and see what really matters
And how to change our ways

Waterways clearer, skies less polluted
New businesses grown from the ashes of the old
Necessity prompting new ideas, reinvention

So, is this virus a friend or foe?

Will we maintain the positive changes?
Once the threat has gone
Or embrace old habits once again

What will you do, how will I be?

Will we still feel united, or go our separate ways?
Is it only extremes that bring us together?
Do you know, do you understand?

What is the virus to you, a glass half empty or a glass half full?

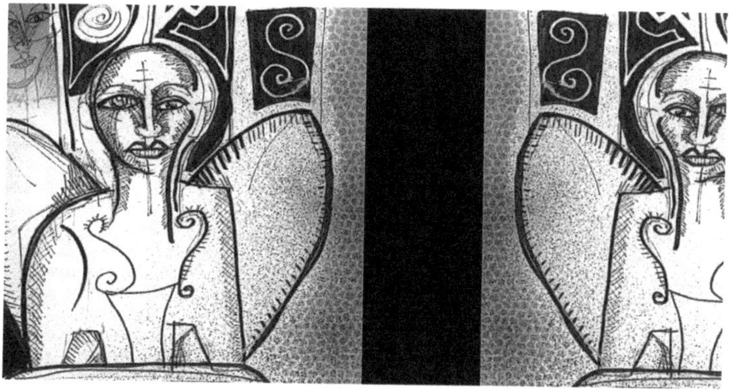

Solitude

Johnnie Dalton

Amid the solitude.
Such delicate words of humour it breeds.
From idle minds it feeds.
While planting doubtful seeds of reality.

Yet so many still fail to believe
The words spoken.
A promise not broken.
Where death is sometimes the token.
Even though we live in fear.
Can the end be near?

In solitude remain.
Break the chain.
At last to be free from the pain.
To live again.
So much knowledge.
Of life.
We will have gained.

London on Lockdown

Carmina Masoliver

bird's-eye view
no people pass
just occasional cars
no tourists taking pictures
no commuters in queues
no football fans flocking
to stadiums, just updates on news
no crowds,
just empty carriages
no funerals,
no marriages
for now,
we wait in homes
like water
simmering on a stove
daily walks
where our hair sways
the end unknown
we countdown days.

Solitaire

Jane Lovell

We don't mention days gone or days left:

longevity is measured in the pyrex
she's had since the 50s,
its crazed surface a frosted window
to a time more comfortable
for both of us,
before I spoilt the order of things.

From her chair in the far room
she gives me directions to the cupboard
with the Denby casserole,
don't use the le creuset,
a wooden spatula from the drawer;
I mustn't use metal
or the good cutlery
or the china teacups stacked like vertebrae
in the dining room,

or the omelette pan.

On the hob is the frying pan that was her mother's,
black as a gypsy's, built for a fire, made
to rest on coals,
older even than my brothers.

From the far room comes the click of solitaire
and the overwhelming flourish of a harp

from the ipad;
electronic angels await her.

There is the patience of the newspaper
as she scratches at the crossword,

and something burgeoning in the papery drifts
of silence,
mathematically, to the power of something unknown,
like sudoku,
when everything suddenly falls into place.

Mitosis.

I stir the jam, damsons splitting into bright pulp,
blisters of boiling sugar,
its brown foam.

Tomorrow I'll make chutney, onion jam.

She stays in the far room.
Every time I leave or enter, I must close the door.
She says, close all the doors,
keep us safe.

London Sleeps

Laura Zuwa Ukpokolo

For the first time in many years,
London slept.
The rare sound of birds chirping
No longer disrupted by the hostile, honking of horns
Or two burly men having a row on the street
The constant groans of the trains halting on tracks eased.
(How had this become the soundtrack we lived by? / an anthem for the modern way of living?)

The steady rhythm of destruction.
Roads were no longer bloated by traffic that congested her scenery,
We watched her longingly from our windows,
Wandering how we were so insatiable,
Now we envied the way the wind would brush against her trees,
Longing - as time stretched lazily into summer,
Possibly…
A message from God? A higher being? Mother nature?
Begging us to slow down
Seeing how universal suffering had given the earth an opportunity to exhale
We never apologised for how we bruised the land that fed us
Instead, we gave flimsy excuses
We could no longer hide behind towering corporate offices
Or squeeze ourself underground, wedged between the armpits of numerous strangers

We never had the time
Now the time had us
In a state of introspection
Wishing back the things we wished away
But we also realised
The jobs of those paid minimum wages
were not so minimal in order for us to survive,
Surgical scrubs were finally recognised as the superhero cloaks they were,
We didn't need to inhale a big mac every two minutes to breathe,
Fast food, fast fashion had finally closed its doors
And the city that never sleeps...

Pressed snooze on the alarm clock.

Escape Route

Karl Nova

I'm indoors
sitting on the floor, bored
acutely aware of squeaking floorboards
above me I wonder what's going on
as the fridge freezer whirs and purrs

Deep in thought
In this moment caught
I want to escape but the world's on pause
in my mind I rewind memories then fast forward
this will never feel normal it's awkward

I'm the sort
to turn things over and over
and turn 'em inside and out, I'm not closer
to cooking up a plot, in my mind's steaming pot
my shawshank redemption is so far off

Time is short
so they say but it feels lengthened
we're sitting here as if it's detention
a lot of tension is whispered from the walls
"books are doors, get out now, don't stall!"

Self-Isolation

Aoife Mannix

Your sleeping face as still
as the nebula reflection
of tree branches in the rainwater
of the blue toy tractor. Your breathing
the coo of wood pigeons, soft as petals
unfurling in the ides of March.
This fear of a glass prison inside a cough.

We are once more alone, time travelling
on the sofa, but gathering our wings
for a short skip through garden sunshine.
You are all look at this zooming in
and out of hairy grass, the daffodil bricks
nodding in a broken mirror. The click
of your surprise. Boy photographer
stepping out of the shadow of sickness.

Though by evening we are back
in the long drink of water as you lose
your voice to fever questions.
I have no answers as the world
shrinks into a screen rolling
with rows of empty shelves
and morning is a long time coming.

Solitude

Seadeta Osmani

Golden are the ornaments of my jail.

The bed is soft and pillows
are dressed in silk.

There is this breeze
caressing me before each sunset,
coming to me through
a brass window.
I can't see the window,
but I know it's there.

My jail is all in carpets,
walls are dressed in curtains,
diamonds reach me
from the ceiling.

If it had a door,
I know the knob would have been golden, too.
But it has none.
No door, no escape.
Running to solitude, in all the fear
but eager to rest my heart,
I lost the door – it fell off
of my shoulders
and I never bothered to
pick it back up.
I thought I would not need it.
I thought I was safe from myself.

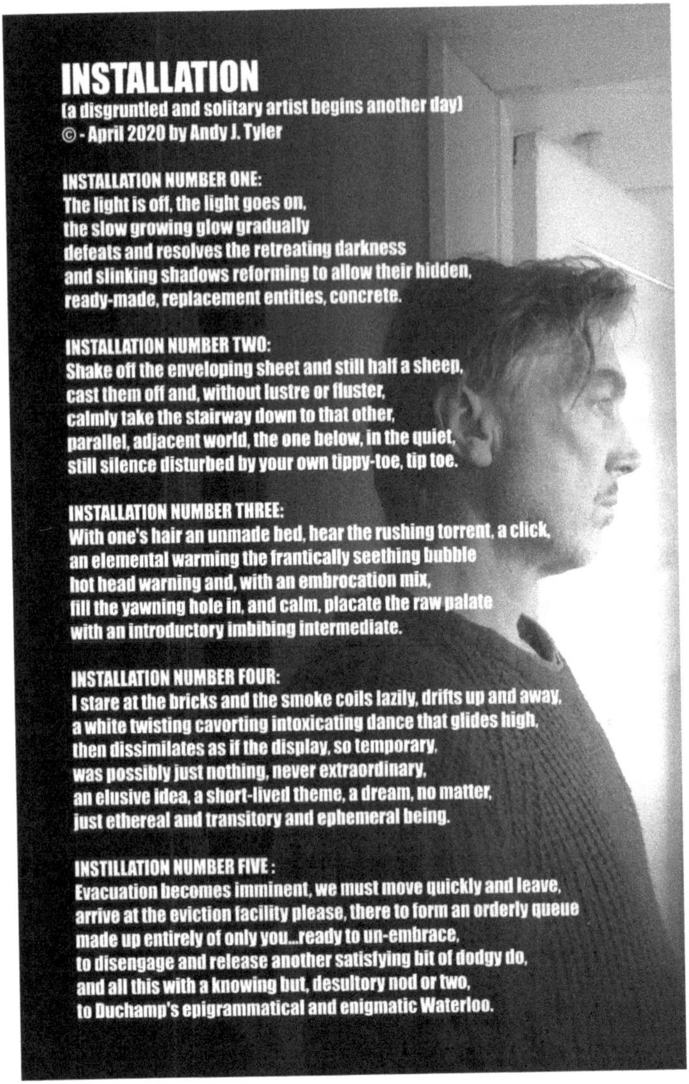

INSTALLATION

(a disgruntled and solitary artist begins another day)
©- April 2020 by Andy J. Tyler

INSTALLATION NUMBER ONE:
The light is off, the light goes on,
the slow growing glow gradually
defeats and resolves the retreating darkness
and slinking shadows reforming to allow their hidden,
ready-made, replacement entities, concrete.

INSTALLATION NUMBER TWO:
Shake off the enveloping sheet and still half a sheep,
cast them off and, without lustre or fluster,
calmly take the stairway down to that other,
parallel, adjacent world, the one below, in the quiet,
still silence disturbed by your own tippy-toe, tip toe.

INSTALLATION NUMBER THREE:
With one's hair an unmade bed, hear the rushing torrent, a click,
an elemental warming the frantically seething bubble
hot head warning and, with an embrocation mix,
fill the yawning hole in, and calm, placate the raw palate
with an introductory imbibing intermediate.

INSTALLATION NUMBER FOUR:
I stare at the bricks and the smoke coils lazily, drifts up and away,
a white twisting cavorting intoxicating dance that glides high,
then dissimilates as if the display, so temporary,
was possibly just nothing, never extraordinary,
an elusive idea, a short-lived theme, a dream, no matter,
just ethereal and transitory and ephemeral being.

INSTILLATION NUMBER FIVE :
Evacuation becomes imminent, we must move quickly and leave,
arrive at the eviction facility please, there to form an orderly queue
made up entirely of only you...ready to un-embrace,
to disengage and release another satisfying bit of dodgy do,
and all this with a knowing but, desultory nod or two,
to Duchamp's epigrammatical and enigmatic Waterloo.

LAND AND SEA

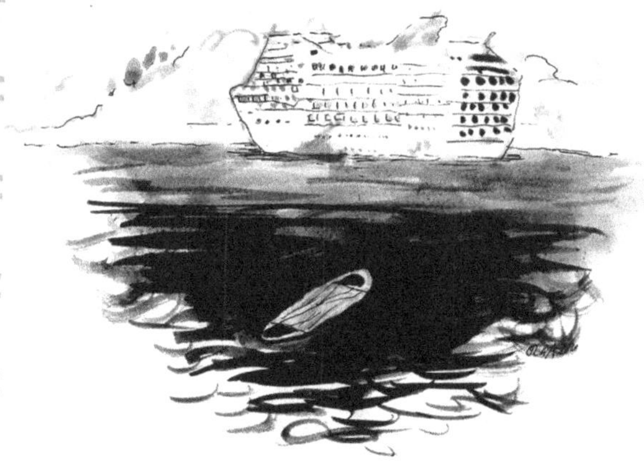

Olga Solabarrieta

Francis H Powell, Clare Reddaway,
Manuella Mavromichalis,
January L'Angelle,
David K MacDonald

New World

Francis H Powell

An angel comes out of the mist
leaving a trail of golden dust
everything glistens and shimmers
awakening to sound of summer
a cloud bursts, as the heavens open
thorny brambles are cut down
replaced by a colourful bloom
and a dash of luring splendour
those heavy chains that weighed us down
are released to the sound of euphoric bliss

As a ship sets sail on a voyage of hope
who wants to take the helm?
A new start, is what we need
A new way of thinking
What we thought is important
is now confined to insignificance
The new Gods are those that cure and heal
The thinkers and philosophers
rule the waves, the skies, the lands we roam

Our leaders have let us down
We have to learn and absorb
we have to find new frontiers
The world has changed
The world is different
Throw out your clutter
Align with planets
cherish the good things we have
those gifts that come from nature

The Longest Journey

Clare Reddaway

She's never been one for the crowded places. The town squares with their fountains and their tourists, the pedestrianised areas thronging with shoppers, the pubs full of drinkers spilling onto the streets. No. She likes the quiet. And the wild spaces. Mountains and moors scratched with heather, rasping at your ankles. Waves crashing on a rocky shore, an empty beach spooling out in front of her tramping boots.

Now, she is inside. She's one of the vulnerable. Her door must stay locked. Death lies just over the threshold, over there, outside.

Her flat is dark. Small. A bad conversion in a Victorian tenement. It smells of basement and of damp. It didn't matter before. It was where she dumped her bags, rested between trips, a stopover place. She never meant it to become her world. The view from her kitchen sink is of the 'courtyard', a pokey dirty space originally designed for coal deliveries, all blackened bricks and dead leaves. There is only a postage stamp of sky.

She feels the sadness creeping in. All the losses. All the regrets. The times when she should have stepped into an embrace but held back, awkward, the times when she should have smiled and said I love you, but was too diffident, the many times when shyness overcame her and the moment was lost forever. And the other times, when she was shunned, or rejected, or harassed, all those times crowd into her head until all she can do is crawl under the covers, curl into a ball and sleep and sleep and sleep.

On the fourth day of sleep she drags herself from bed to bathroom and then to kettle and as she waits for it to boil, she looks out into the courtyard. Prison yard, she thinks. The high walls, the patch of sky. There's a bin bag, blown in from the street, caught in the drain. If it rains, that'll flood, she thinks. She makes herself unlock the door, push hard and step out, in her flipflops, into the air. It's dank and dark of course, but it is not the rank air of her bedroom and there is light, filtering down.

She tugs at the bin bag, frees the drain, then, like a prisoner, she steps along the edge of the yard. Ten steps. She runs her fingertips over the rough texture of the red brick. Ten more steps across the back, then ten again, and ten back to the door. A square, of forty steps. A step is about two and a half feet. Two thousand steps makes one mile, ten thousand is five miles. She knows this. This is enough.

On that first day she walks around the area five times. The air fills her lungs and although she goes back to her bed and retreats into the dark her head is beginning to fill with other images, with other thoughts, and when she wakes the next morning she gets straight out of bed. She has a plan.

She finds the old tin of white paint that is hidden at the back of a cupboard and a paint brush that has hardened with lack of use. She levers open the tin and there is plenty of paint, plenty as she sloshes it on the walls of the area, plenty to make it white. It doesn't matter that the paint splatters on the ground, and it doesn't matter that it might peel off in a few months or become stained green with mould. What matters is that now the walls are bright and white and she has a canvas.

She finds her Ordinance Survey maps. She chooses one to begin. It is her favourite. She steps out into the courtyard. She starts at the pub in the village and walks through three fields until she gets to the edge of the moor. She climbs up the steep slope, her feet finding footholds in the rocky footpath. She meets the burn and puts her hand into the peaty water, splashing her face to cool it. She doesn't smell the new paint now, but the fragrance of heather, coming into bloom, the coconut scent of yellow gorse and the crystal clean air of the hilltop.

That morning her limbs feel heavy and tired from the exercise but her brain feels sharper than it has for days. She feels the need to mark her walk, to record it, as a prisoner might. She has oil paints, bought for a project long discarded. Standing in front of the shining white walls, she paints the new purple blush of the heather which covers the moor. The second day is an oak tree, stunted and bent by the wind. The third day she paints a hare, guarding its leveret in the grass.

By the third week she looks out of her kitchen window to a wild space, thronging with life, with green, with mountains, with birds, with rocks and caves, with sky. She looks out into a landscape of freedom.

She rings her mother.

"Hi Mum," she says. "I've been on the longest journey."

Golden Talons

Manuella Mavromichalis

At night I step out from within my walls
I place the golden talons of Zeus' eagles upon my fingers
And tear through the veil – into the dreaming
I buckle Hermes' winged sandals upon my feet and step over
To the place between the mundane and the wild
Between the past, present and future
Between the hard light of day and the gauze of night
And the world beyond the veil – envelops me

I am transported to the mountains of Delphi,
Back to the narcotic scent of jasmine, overripe figs
 and wild oregano
Salt spray coated skin
The calling song of the crickets
Black pine saplings bowing to the wind
Up the sacred path, across the mountain,
Down the valley below,
Thousands of olive trees,
The sea an azure backdrop to the earthy greens
and mottled browns.
I am the Oracle
Holding audience, as Apollo's whispered riddles caress my ear
I take in the fumes rising up from the chasm,
Through the Omphalos, brushing my thighs
Over my breasts
And surrender to ecstasy and delirium

I am at the temple of Hera in my beloved Samos,
Sweet Samian wine upon my lips, under my tongue
Immersed in the ice-cold waters of Ireon,
My skin – goose flesh
The moon, full and silver
Water nymphs calling me deeper and further from the shore
Our limbs tangled, our exchanged breaths – our life force
The Sirens' song calls to us, but we will not succumb to it,
For we have found our own hymn to worship to
We let the cool and warm currents wash over our skin
And invite wild abandonment and elation to consume us

I am on the rock of Aphrodite
Singing softly to myself,
The syllables of the Greek language twisting around my tongue,
The vowels filling my mouth.
Their melody evoking all the senses with its cadence.
The call of a lover serenading her heart's passion,
The rhythmic whooshing of the waves against the shore,
The swaying of the branches of the bergamot tree
Showering its blossoms upon the earth,
Anointing everything it touches with its gentle brush and pungent aroma.

These walls cannot contain me
As long as poetry resounds within me
As long as myths and stories entwine with my every thought
As long as the gods reside within the temple that is me
As long as frescoes, icons, sculptures and mosaic adorn me
As long as I imbue the flavours of my ancestors and our history
As long as incense perfumes my hallowed spaces

My spirit is indomitable and light
It glides and roams wherever it wills
For you cannot cage nor chain that which is free

At night I step out from within my walls
I place the golden talons of Zeus' eagles upon my fingers
And tear through the veil – into the dreaming

Princess of the Sea

January L'Angelle

Based on the tragedy that occurred on the Diamond Princess cruise during the pandemic.

She was a Princess, known to all
This Princess, would soon take a fall
At first glance, she was breathtaking,
sparkling, but awaiting no king.

Tricking guests with her royal fanfare,
swallowing them in the lion's lair
Inviting them each into her fold
Feeling so regal, the tale is told.

Subjects lulled like sheep, to their room
Unsuspecting the viral doom
Grasping the castles toxic rail
They readied themselves to set sail.

The Princess invited all to dine
Most all partook in a glass of wine
The subjects sat shoulder to shoulder
The evil lurked bolder and bolder.

Laughter was heard throughout dinner
Was the enemy the winner?
He dropped his poison like an opus
It smothered the weakest among us.

Off to bed went all the infected,
rapidly the aged descended
Poisoned like hemlock in days of yore,
the frail, the first to fall to the floor.

A slain man in my direction, toward
Where's the enemy… to point my sword?
I can't fight what my eyes don't see
Death befalls a man so quickly.

The Princess looks for safe harbor
And drifts about… who'll help her?
When craving for human touch,
no more need for the wanderlust.

The princess would have many die
To those lost we must say goodbye.

Why the sea?

David K MacDonald

These salty sailors, their brave facade
To live on earth
Where foot is fine
The sea no place to tread
No riches by the air divine

Its rolling mass
Its constant sway
Its creatures vast
Its darkness grey
Its gleaming gift
Its wondrous scent
Its rape, the price of man's betray

Why kill this place
Where bodies lie
Why oil the arms
For soft embrace
Why make it sick
And watch in awe
The spray its tears to cry

Why pray for souls and sigh
All it swallows
All its anger
Why can't we see
It's only on its grace we sail

No natural place for you and me
But turn it will
And in its churning mass
Its boil of blood
Will cry
Why me?
Why the sea?

DIFFERENT PERSPECTIVES

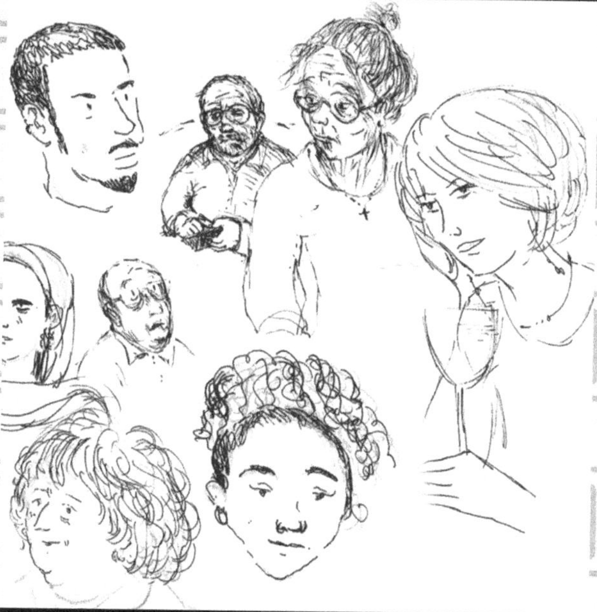

Suki Spangles, Camilla Nelson, Gail Meath, B. Lynn Goodwin, Toby Campion (USA), Francis H Powell, Roy Duffield, Derek Thompson, D.L. Lang, Arti Rai, Rosie Carick, Armand Ruhlman, Nina Zee(vancevic), Harry Weiss Jones, Peter Finch, Stewart Taylor, Alun Robert, Muni Subhradip Chakraborty, Rhian Edwards, Ciara MacLaverty, Katrina Naomi, Alison Brackenbury, Sue Hardy-Dawson, A.F. Harrold, Lynne Reid Banks, Paul Matthews, Marcus Christopherson, Trevor Millum, Mark Heathcote, Ashish Kapoor, Rita Rana, Ariadne Radi Cor, Magi Gibson, Mark Blickley

A Stranger Takes Your Hand

Suki Spangles

A stranger holds your hand
Grips it tightly
They are just holding on
to your hand
They don't want anything from you
The stranger doesn't want to hurt you
The stranger is giving something to you
And you most likely won't see them again.

Surfacing

Camilla Nelson

Glittering daisy fronds show no end of malice.

Grasses claw & slice.   The wood

fluffs unevenly into life.   A green mattress

fans into a peacock   canopy.

Shuffling blackthorns   caterpillar the boundary.

You are beside me still   in this uneven tension

& I love you for it.

I Am a Colour

Gail Meath

I can fade into the background without notice
or stand brightly alone for the world to see.

Serene shades of blue are my warmth and compassion,
deep shades like midnight hold all of my dreams.
Dark mixtures of green grip my fears and defenses,
which stop me from reaching all that I can be.

The glitter of gold emits courage and honesty,
Stark yellow streaks keep my daring at bay.
Flavors of orange foretell sunshine or rain,
yet blood red forewarns to keep out of my way.

Purple is flashy, my love for adventure.
Violet portrays my adoration for fun.
And when I get lost in the swirl of it all,
brown is resistant and settles me down.

I am color. A visual image with many hues.
I am never black, never white and never gray.

Living in a Dystopian World (Fiction Letter)

B. Lynn Goodwin

The only time I ever lived in a dystopian world was back in 2020 during the time of the Corona Virus. While sheltering-in-place, I only went out to walk Eddie McPuppers. I worried about all of you. I was tutoring a 14-year-old boy and often wondered, as I watched him compete and thrive, if you were doing the same.

That was the year that your Great Uncle Richard almost had to lay-off all his employees, including two sons and a grandson. That was the only time he stopped holding church services, although he planned to do them online after a couple weeks. It was a time when gas prices dropped and I went for three weeks without filling my tank.

My hair got grey at the roots. It became shapeless. I did not care. Why care when the only person I saw was my husby and he didn't notice my hair? He didn't lose interest in other things, but I digress.

So what made the world dystopian? Work was forbidden for almost everyone who was not a part of the medical community or an essential service. Social distancing required us to stay 6 feet apart. Hand sanitizers were everywhere and at the bank, there was a manager designated to make sure everyone used it.

Roads were relatively empty. Investments dipped. But the overlying feeling was that no one knew what the enemy was or what the future held. We were very afraid that we would never return to the normal we had known at the beginning of the year when our President insisted that the Corona Virus was the new hoax. I'm sure you've studied the Trump era, and I wonder how much your textbooks, if you still use those, cleaned it up. But that's a subject for another letter.

I am leaving this as part of a legacy that I hope you'll see someday. If not, you'll hear about this life changing time from others, and maybe you'll have the perspective to see it in a light that we missed while we were living through it. Whatever happens, I give you love and light and hope that you never deny the realities that touch you.

What She Wanted Most... (Fiction Reflection)

B. Lynn Goodwin

What she wanted most of all was peace. Her head rang despite the fact that there was nothing but a little white noise in her condo. Maybe her head rang from an invisible throbbing in her ears or her brain drowning out the sounds of diagnosis and death.

Covid-19 didn't really affect her. She didn't know anyone who'd caught it. Her husband was out in the world daily, but she hadn't even been to a grocery store in over a week. She used to watch the news, but now her mind blocked anything that wasn't fiction or a tangible situation that she had some control over. The outside world was crumbling, and that's why she stayed inside. She wanted to live in peace-the way she did before the world went wonky.

If she couldn't have peace, she'd settle for a back button that worked on real life. Something that would take her back to a time before Covid-19, even she spent too much time commuting back then and every little mistake felt like a major failure. That was before life and death could be measured in a misdirected breath. When did breathing become lethal?

All her life she lived with allergies that afflicted her respiratory system whenever blossoms appeared and new grass sprouted. That was happening again, as if the world would go on whether she was in it or not.

How could she be in danger? She stayed inside, washed her hands, and was slipping into an emotional whirlpool. That would be safe as long as no one spit in it, right?

Peace was such an abstract thing. She should ask for

ventilators, masks, and an end to the re-infection rate. No more of this random cleansing of the population. Not on her watch. Like she had a watch or any influence at all on the things that meant life or death these days.

If this were her last day on earth, what would she want to do? If she couldn't answer the question, it couldn't be her last day. Logic like that lived in the old world. She still hadn't found the Rules of Survival in this altered world that nibbled away at her outer brain cells.

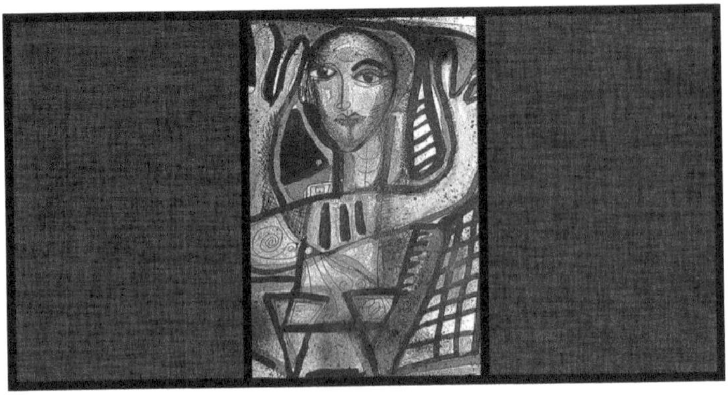

Living Trust

Toby Campion (U.S.)

By the powers within me
    And in full possession
Of my impermanence,
    I hereby assign and bequeath

Unto my shoes, my feet;
    Unto my hat, my head;
Unto my wife, my heart;
    Unto this day, my life.

I nominate my children
    To be themselves in toto,
No bond but love, freely
    Given, full benefits.

God Almighty shall be
    The trustee of my estate,
Mother Earth disposing
    Of the rest and residue.

Seabird

Roy Duffield

a life
alone
asleep and
a wake
on a bed of memory-less
foam
and waves
to no-one
where nothing
is ever the same
and everything
always looks the same
not a soul
but a sole
in sight
no solid
soil
to lay my feet
'til we land on land
to mate
and meet
and share
for a moment and
forever
our lonely fate.

How Far Pluto is from the Sun

Roy Duffield

How far you are
from the Sun
pre-1931.
They're completely unaware.
They don't even know you're there
as you set out
on your longest journey yet
we'll never be this close again
cut off
behind a wall
of black-out paint
three billion miles thick
and counting…
and just out of reach
frozen through
−218 degrees
and counting…
of insufficient mass
and far too far
from anything else
(four billion miles now
and still counting…)
for anything else
to be moved
by the pull of your gravity
as you fall away
exponentially
faster
faster
than this message could ever follow

lost
in silence
(zero decibels
but now who's counting?)
They taught us in Science
to know
but never to understand.

RSVP

Derek Thompson

Bernard sat in the library in his usual chair, reading his newspaper, poised over the thick rings around the job ads. Here and there he'd underlined some of the key words, the way he always did: *conscientious, flexible, interpersonal skills.* It hadn't taken long to decipher the limited vocabulary of the jobs market. The terminology was as much about conferring status on the post itself as it was about getting the right candidates.

Writing, Bernard considered as he scratched a pen mark beneath *strategic,* exalted both the writer and the reader. All were enriched by the majesty of language – the commonplace rendered wondrous.

Eyes closed, he saw the words fluttering before him – not just their words, but the ones he would craft together in reply, like a lover's response. For every motif in print, he would sift through the treasure trove of his own mental thesaurus, or if he was really stymied – the one in the reference section.

For *conscientious*, he would write *dedicated* or maybe *hardworking; flexible* would muster *adaptable* at first, which he'd perhaps refine to *multi-skilled* or *able to embrace change* – as the situation dictated. *Interpersonal skills,* he'd likely break down into *good listener* and *an effective communicator.*

Bernard folded his paper and started to dream about the crisp, lined sheets he always used for writing job applications longhand. He could almost hear the crick, crick of the pencil sharpener as he set to work – the first draft always in 2B pencil.

Last month had been a particularly good month for replies and interview offers. And of course, it didn't end there. Not by any means. There were letters of polite decline to send on – some indicating an alternative job offer and others hinting at a family tragedy or untoward circumstances. If he were to receive a condolence card in response – and it sometimes happened that way – he always saved it and added it to his collection.

It was always nice to receive a letter. Sometimes, when the letters were so darn polite and welcoming, it almost made him wish he were qualified for the job and could attend the interview. But mostly, it was nice to receive a letter, and nicer still to be appreciated.

We Long

D.L. Lang

Do you remember what it was like before the world shut down?
Do you remember how we crowded into our favorite bar
to be serenaded are the sweet symphony of guitars?
Do you remember how exciting it was to sit in the theater
surrounded by complete strangers enjoying the same film?

Now we sit alone accompanied only by the radio,
and wonder if we will ever see our friends again.
We long to feel their presence, to be held in their arms,
to hear the sound of their laughter. Oh, dear friends!

Isolation nibbles on a lonely heart left unfulfilled.
There is a hunger raging deep inside our souls.
We long for community. We long for connection.

So many souls are taking their final journey
unaccompanied by sacred rituals of the past
meant to comfort those of us left behind.

We long to be able to comfort one another,
and ride the waves of communal sustenance,
but we stand disconnected, threadbare,
uncertain of what shall come next,
searching for the buoyancy of hope.

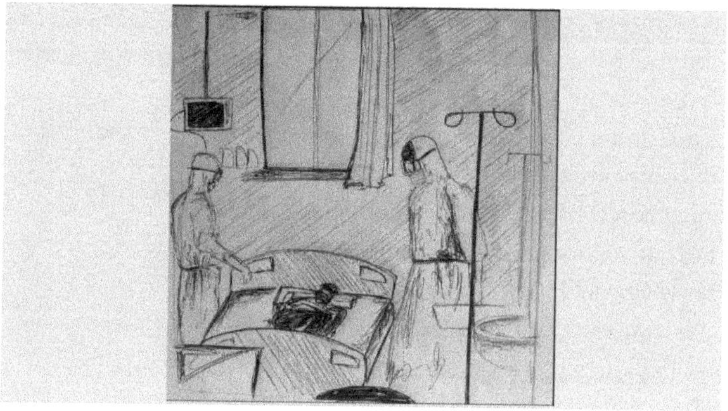

When Corona

Arti Rai

When the mischievous Corona
walks down naked on the streets
of gorgeous world or seeps into
gracious humans through little
nostrils or openings of beautiful
eyes and catchy wise ears,
a terror strikes and a cold shiver knocks
down the spine, sickness sounds high.
Folks suddenly wash their hands they
never had done before so madly.
Quarantine becomes the usage of
the time, husbands and wives sort out their matters over many
cups of teas and coffees at breakfast.
Many couples, it came in The Print,
fight unto divorces for such closeness
as this had never happened before.
Children yell and dance for schools have closed at once, no
exams, no fear of failing merry life begins out of the blue.

Aeroplanes rest drooping faces in
the cool hangers and roads have found some hibernation, a relief
free from the thumping footfalls.
Ye, Corona you are cute! Say the birds flying free in the
uncompetitive sky
air is bereft of venom and scorching
heat of carbon trash. So clear a sky!
How Corona! How? Why did you do so!
Are you a warning to unrest humans
or just a signal, a flash of horrid future.
Hey, corona it's enough,go , take your
course in mysterious woods go or
your death warrant would be issued.
Corona! Take it as a warning!
Man has overcome all in all the ages
Life goes on! You know it well!

16 wks

Rosie Carick

A flutter
From the inside out
Left to right.
A flickering message
In one
(tap tap)
And with that
And no more
I knew you were there
I knew you were mine
And that we were alright.

Forth from My Cave

Armand Ruhlman

Today, I ventured forth from my cave into the East Village landscape...

which now looks and feels like a netherworld from a very bad dream...

a quite shocking experience to be surrounded by a kind of desolation and abandonment as I walked through areas of the neighborhood that were usually overflowing with a motley mix of residents and visitors...

artists, students, trust funders, elderly retirees, teenage skateboarders, winos, bums, beggars, bubble-headed bimbos from the hinterlands of New Jersey, college kids, fraternity Bro's looking to get wasted in one of the gazillion bars, dogs on leashes, babies in carriages, young couples seeking a future, old couples trying to remember what they thought the future might be...Hebrews, Arabs, Muslims, Hindus, Irish, French, Indian, Chinese, Mexicans, Russians (look, is that Putin, in the East Village?)...and a few Anglo-Saxons - from Quebec?...and last but least, a middle-aged former Catholic Schoolboy from N'awlins (which is sinking into the sea) currently narrating this re-telling...

my simple, even humble objective was to go to the grocery store for a few carrots and a can of beans – to go with my cold leftovers of limp spaghetti and even limper Romaine lettuce...

waiting – with everyone about 6 feet apart – in line for admittance to the emporium...

then wallowing in paranoia once inside the store as I try to maintain appropriate social distancing while surrounded by a new breed of creature...

at least a new bred to me...in the age of Trump and the virus....in the age of a used car salesman being put in charge of the earth as the world comes to an end...

this new breed of creature – which apparently has been hiding from me in plain sight – emerges whenever I leave my apartment...

emerges to either surrounded me or come dangerously close to violating my sacred space – sacred to me, anyway – as I keep to myself and attempt to maneuver down the sidewalks of New York...

this creature – young, old, rich poor, white, black, brown, yellow, red, or green(?) – seems to have been taking in a totally different reality from the daily bouts of horrible news that I've been receiving...

horrible news about the infections and deaths and lack of testing and all of that jazz – to go with the massive explosion of lies and the resulting distrust of our so-called leaders...

(if the Martians landed and demanded my leader(?) would I offer him up the alien beings...why not...?)

thus, this new breed of creature seems to move with impunity through the surrounding environs...

impunity, arrogance, selfishness – and surely aloofness – regarding the possible consequences of being infected by the virus from another, less fortunate, creature...

or passing it on as some kind of asymptomatic carrier of the damn thing...

and this new breed of creature, infected with an attitude of: make way, here I come...almost reminds me of a miniature balloon from the Macy's thanksgiving day parade that has escaped and is steadily marauding its way across the landscape... expecting everyone to move, jump, dive, twist, and turn out of the way of this imperial(?) ass(?) who feels free to speak, breathe, exhale, and god knows what upon the surrounding sea of desperate souls looking for the last roll of bathroom tissue in the local emporium...damn, I never thought the local grocery store could be a journey through the depths of hell. And let's not even think about the checkout counter.

Corona beer diaries

Nina Zee(vancevic)

I saw myself shaking and trembling while crossing the street,
then I saw a man stepping 2 meters away from me as he saw me both of us shaking and trembling in the street.
I quickly went back home and started reading the DECAMERON.

In fact, I grew up in a family which sadly, forbid me to be weak. This morning, as a local doctor has come to see me I noticed how tired he was. I asked him if he was OK, to which he said "Oh, if you had only known how I'd feel!"

I said I knew exactly how he felt. He said "How's so?"

I said I remember my mother telling me the story of when she was 19 and the first year student of Medicine, she was taken to Sremski Front. It was like the battle at Stalingrad, I explained, to which the doc said "WOW!"

So this young girl (my mom) was ordered to make an arbitrary choice. Her superior was walking with them (the trainees) through the field filled with the wounded and the dying and right there, my mom had to make a very quick choice whether to help one person and let the other one die. The supervisor had ordered them not to examine a soldier longer than 45 seconds. There, they would have detected if he was to be'helped' by the medical staff or it was simply too late to do anything for him.

The first group of soldiers which could be helped and taken away was GROUP A. The second, which was totally helpless and forlorn, was GROUP B. My mother remembered that it was not THAT difficult to stay awake without food or sleep for 10 days and 10 nights working endlessly at Sremski field but the heaviest thing was to be the judge and decide who was going to be saved and who was going to die. Mom said that she would never forget the eyes of the dying and that all of them were only calling "mother, mother help me!"

"WOW!" exclaimed my visiting doctor again "This is how I feel right now – the war medicine is the heaviest branch of them all.."

"So, dear doc, can YOU tell me where would you put my case- into group A ...or group B?" I asked lightly.

You just sleep and take paracetamol and after 2-3 weeks you'll be ok."

I am quite OK, in fact, as long as I don't have to make decisions and give orders or indictments about who is to live and who's to die..

Corona beer diaries 2

If I didn't have to go to the toilet every 10 to 15 minutes, this quarantine would even be fun! However, every picture has its frame, every picture tells a story: there is a story where the most idiotic people call to ask me (they are sweet I guess) how I feel. I cough and sneeze and spit blood through my mouth and through nostrils – the skin tissue ripped open – is this THE one which Poe called 'the Mask of Red Death'?

I don't know.. have been through so many of them, even from the times when they changed DNA in my cells (2008) and I saw all people in the form of the angelic visions – in fact, they were very ordinary, all of them – except for an old witch. This prophetess à la Nostradamus, was actually giving a crystal ball clairvoyant session when Marc-Louis brought me to her spooky place.

As soon as I entered the room, the prophetess exclaimed "WHO is ,or rather who was a Buddhist nun among you here ?"

"It's me, it's me", I yelled.

"And who used to be a painter in her previous life?", she continued.

"It's me, it's me", I tweeted again.

"I see you entirely burnt", she said, "you are covered with ashes- but like a phoenix", she continued, "YOU will rise from the ashes!"

I was so grateful to hear her soothing bullshit. The chemotherapy had burnt all my cells and then, my DNA was changed entirely so that I could live like a bionic woman, and as far as I go, that was fine for me. That was 12 years ago.

This time around I appeared even more belligerent, as my trip to Kerala in 2014 , when I'd caught malaria again, taught me that one could die and resurrect several times.

I will challenge this man-made virus, this lousy convention again invented by an even lousier scientist whose nose was dripping with coke and his own experiment -- so why burn my throat and my stomach so drastically now? NO ONE could convince me that this batman was using bats - for his batty business! There must have been something more powerful at his hand. And us humans - we were in this affair all alone - offered to the mercy of bad commerce and distant trade.

Several leaders were competing all over the world in their endeavor to open several V.I. markets, in order to erase the surplus of humans on earth, as just VERY few computer educated jocks were supposed to work from home. I mean, to work. And the rest of us were not supposed to work - as we were duly supposed to die. Or just try to die, which was fine with me, but as usual, in my case that was very very bad timing. (Do I really sound like that scumbag Burroughs?)

What about that book of essays on FILM? Unfinished.

What about my BOOK Project on Theater? Not achieved yet.. And the translations. And some new violin scores...? That goes endless.

OK, I take a deep breath, time to meditate in solitude again. For us, creatures of the air (Zodiac Air Sign) and birds, pterodactyls, butterflies, ghosts witches, bubbles of all sorts, it is so darn difficult not to be able to deeply inhale the air.. Just that little..

I take a deep breath: One.. TWO.. THREE, auch auch, cough and spit again. There, where a lung was, it's an open window, a sort of a burnt hole. Dark Star, by Ziggy Stardust, speckles of white chlorochyde dust..

Corona beer diaries 3

for my friend Virna T.

I have just returned from the visit to a doctor B. He refused to give me the test as he observed my symptoms.

"Aha, you answered all my question positively, so, take the prescription against this ailment and go to the pharmacy. Stay in bed for two weeks and call me back." He must had been scared of any further visit.

At the pharmacy next to my quarantined home, all the pharmacists were protected by a glass shield. A young fellow who was particularly caring announced "Do not worry, just take the medication and go back home safely, in two weeks you will develop the antibodies and you will be OK!"

I went back home, but when I looked into my mirror, my face was as white as Alexanriane Sarane's one day before he died in hospital. However, on that last day of his life, he was cool and kind and loving, professional above all – to write a blurb for my book 'Under the Sign of Cyber Cybele'. What a bright example of how a poet should behave!

Then numerous phone calls have started to flood in. Four of my former husbands have called. Basically they all had to say the same thing.

Call no. 1:

The snazzy and soft voice of my number one has declared: "Oh, I just wanted to see how you are doing.. I meant to tell you.. hmm, I've always wanted to tell you that I have always loved you and cared for you from the start... This is not a final call, but I just want you to know- I apologize for everything."

YES, I said, "What for, sweety?"

"Well, if I had said or done anything wrong to you.. Just to tell you know how much I love you."

"Oh, thank YOU! I love you too!"

Call no. 2:

"Hi! You haven't heard from me for a while," an ever dynamic voice of husband no.2 exclaimed, "that's because I've been so busy, so busy dealing with all these insane people, however, you know that I love you, right ? I've always loved you, and even now, as of this very moment, if you ever wanted to come back to me, you know my door, that is my heart, is always open, how do you feel?"

"Fine", I answered. "A bit tired, but I'll be OK."

"You'd better be OK," he added, "you know we are supposed to meet in London in 3 months. That gives you enough time to recover... this is just to tell you...I apologize for everything !"

"YES," I said, "what for, sweety?"

"Well, if I had said or done anything wrong to you. Just to tell you know how much I love you."

"Oh, thank YOU ! I love you too !"

Call no. 3:

"Hello, my dearest Queen of Hearts!"The exhuberant voice of no.3 was penetrating my ear through the excellent receiver of my iphone.

"I'm calling you as I have noticed that you posted some alarming notices on your Facebook page. Is it all true? What's wrong with your health now?" And not allowing me for a second to respond to his numerous questions, he continued, " I hope that you clean your environment, and I DO hope that your son is helping you a bit, that is, I hope that he is well, safe and sound."

"Everyone is ok over here," I respond, "and I truly hope that YOU take care of yourself as your health has been ever fragile ever since.."

"Ohhh," he continued "this is just to tell you...I apologize for everything. !"

"YES," I said, "what for, sweety?"

"Well, if I had said or done anything wrong to you. Just to tell you know how much I love you."

"Oh, thank YOU! I love you too !" I added and wished him good evening, morning time that it was on my side of the planet.

Call no. 4:

"Hello... yes, it's ME! No one else but your silly Mini-me who has been really worried…" I interrupted him: "about the state of the planet in general and my health in particular?"

"There you go!" he answered and having detected these tired overtones in my voice, he continued "Do these doctors do anything good for you over there?"

"Oh, yes, they do," I replied, "but they must be really overworked and awfully exhausted themselves, as this huge epidemic advances.. and my dear, HOW ARE YOU ?"

"YES I KNOW," he, the most reasonable of them four replied, "see, I am a bit on a sickly side too...and my sister is even in a worse condition than I am right now.. but .. this is just to tell you...I apologize for everything!"

"YES," I said, "what for, sweety?"

"Well, if I had said or done anything wrong to you. Just to tell you know how much I love you."

"Oh, thank YOU! I love you too!"

I had no further strength to continue the conversation, as also all these calls appeared a bit repetitive to me. I could not even remember why I had ever parted from J. or even K. for that matter, whereas T. and M. were plainly not compatible with me, but sweet that they all called almost at the same time! The road of human soul is so winding and unpredictable. This time I also refused to believe that they called in order to redeem their own spiritual selves from darkness - it will be OK, now that all of us walked along that steep path of forgiveness.

I went back to my bed and turned the radio on. The Heroic symphony boomed from it; all of us need that extra encouragement, from time to time.

Reflections wrought out of Covid Quarantine

Harry Weiss Jones

One single second split by a frozen shock
as dream chimes strike a molten rock at
now just 5 to human decency.
Set alight with fresh sensation (can it be anticipation?!)
that tears straight through a dull blank stare
of a cynic's boredom; that induced this comatose,
    faithless, reverie.
But, against the grain of the usual strain, compassion's single
tear fell, in torrents and left me drenched, ice cold,
but then doused with boiling thunder,
finally wrenched and roused from a malaise soaked slumber.
That ice cold jolt caressed with warm surprise
a long-deserved assault, that awoke all three of my eyes-
though, I must confess, I'd long since surmised
that all my spirit stone dead, cured and salted lies
served up upon a table.

But still every facet long since shattered
could show the gazer how he got so battered
routine made mince-meant of all that mattered
until resigned to resignation's solitude, he sought victory
    in defeat.
Showing what he saw was truly all it seems;
A generation comforted by memes, not dreams;
in the shape of art enjoyed at a pace of fools
and with ambitions far the lesser.
A simian heart and biological tools

yet with a logic-defying processor
that houses mind's infinite vastness;
but its value pails beside a phone's chic, shiny sharpness
stuck like stigmata to our palm.
Surely tepid stimulation could do no harm?
Why should eyes be made of water and our memories
spoke aloud?
Nature's sighs at gifts we've brought her-
a much less nourishing Apple and its subterranean
dwelling Cloud.
A cloud which launches, not Helen's ships, but
10 thousand falsely filtered faces;
running from envy to envy in online races.
Eternal self in an eternal ether.
Are we so keen to put paid to death that we're forgetting
that we live?

All this beauty shared for ugly reasons, accumulates to merge
the seasons and so one by one we join legions
monetising all we are.
Raping reality with unreal pictures
escaping life's banality with far more banal fixtures:
myriad vapid space-set rom-coms
and the rapid race to get yet more mod-cons
hides the fact our only evolution
is that our blood's now pumped by stone.
Isolation and boredom strangling,
on death's precipice we feel we all are dangling;
yet notice how there's much less petty wrangling,
now there's actual reasons for that anxious groan.
We've spun imagined profit from but have forgot to taste
the heavenly fruit our ancestral dreams have sown.

A creeping, nearly universal worry
(forced to halt our daily ant-like scurry)
could bind a generation who exchanged calm for hurry
until a plague made the truest gifts of life be known.

What For?

Peter Finch

Thrill
Glory on trains
Difficulty surmounted
Fixing the sliding
Identity
Small fame
Many lights no lights sheets of darkness specks of rain
Great renown like a man with arms
with a box file that runs for days
Folk melody
Rays
Unexpected victory
Parts one to twenty-eight (1-28)
Twenty-nine

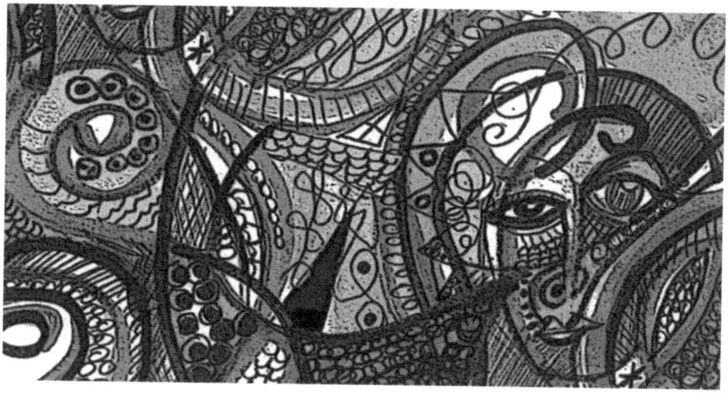

Dreams

Stewart Taylor

I've had some unusual dreams of late,
some of them seem quite real,
like pedalling the path to my granddad's gate
on a bike with just one wheel.
No Natural Law in this dreamlike state
and nothing much changes when I'm awake.
I've had some unusual dreams of late.
Some of them seem quite real.

At A Distance

Alun Robert

At least there's some shelter
in the doorway that once was Woolies
from wind
from rain
from passing feral youth

for I'm on my own
with my Staffy for safety
isolated from the rat race
isolated from the virus
keeping most off the streets

apart from the local charity
of kindly blue rinses
with food parcels
with comfort
who visit most days

so the virus can't catch me
for I'm social distancing
feeling like a leper though
feeling ill from a life style
condemned by most

but at least May is warmer
no more shivers
no more wondering
if I'll have frozen by morning
to die here ignored

by passing feral youth
by wind
by rain
in the doorway that once was Woolies
where there's only isolation.

Joy and Sorrow

Muni Subhradip Chakraborty

When splashes of rains talk to the window pane --
And greener the grass doth look,
When the white white mist; spurs up with a twist,
More silent seemes the brook.

A butterfly; under the leaf so shy,
Looks at the rain with mirth,
A secret splendour, blissful and tender,
In her heart took its birth.

For ages and years we have witnessed here;
The joy that surrounds us:
Through all our pains, through shine and rains;
We conquer the spell of tears 'round us.

In each and every grain of earth, a mark of sorrow resides,
But its twin sister mirth, no matter what, is always by its side.

Forever Parked

Rhian Edwards

Are those the Sunday bells I hear, as clear
as themselves? In ten years of Sunnyside
living, my ears never made your acquaintance.
Is it a renegade bell-ringer, ticking off
the bucket list at a congregationless service?

Never have I inhabited the outside
world of my back garden like this,
under pandemic house arrest,
in the thick of a spring
that is outdoing itself.

My decking has become the French Riviera.
My postage stamp garden is now a playroom,
an obstacle course, a classroom.
The water table and sandpit
a Center Parcs for Barbie.

I've decluttered my shed not once,
but twice. The decorator's table
is forever assembled, paint-splattered,
Play-doh caked. The push bikes
dusted off, tyres resuscitated.

Regard the latest addition of the fire pit.
How it devoured the Christmas tree
that leaned like a drunk, propped up
between the rotting Wendy House
and the freshly varnished fencing.

Is it my imagination or are there
more butterflies, bees, birdsong?
The picnic blanket is a magic carpet,
forever parked, unless the journeys
are essential, but aren't they, always?

Not Really About Snow

Katrina Naomi

It lay there, somewhere between Paddington
and home. My yellow suitcase and I
travelled. I listened to Alice Oswald,
Sasha Dugdale, Sean O'Brien, their certain,
warmed voices, floating
from left ear to right, all that machinery
between. The voices found their frequencies
through the flurries. Each spoke – privately, it seemed –
of a long-dead poet, one I'd never truly met
on the page. I stared out into the dark, knowing
the snow was present only at stations.
It seemed to huddle there, in half-illumination,
as if waiting to board. Between times,
there was my profile, listening, and those earrings
– lobes glowing with red plastic roses –
which didn't quite match my cardy.
There was no one to notice; the carriage as quiet as snow
falling upwards. A reflection is never what a person looks like.
A podcast captures an echo of a person's knowledge.
Yet that night, alone in the empty carriage
but for the voices and for Keats, journeying
for seven hours, I knew my luck. I had a tray
of sushi, the chopsticks crossing themselves,
ginger beer. I felt enchanted with ideas,
neurons sparking towards each other. The carriage
was almost cosy, yesterday's clothes –
their acridity – contained in the case
at my feet, London still wrapped around its wheels.

The drifts of snow out there condensing
like memory before it washes out. But for now,
I had everything. I knew my lover
would be waiting for me on the platform.
I had a home to go to. And I felt blessed.

Flash: remembered in lockdown

Alison Brackenbury

In Kenya, to bleached branch it came,
noon's bird, Malachite kingfisher.
Even the broad beak borrowed flame.

At Rousham – was the Cherwell there? –
with friends who, later, trekked through hell,
sun's amber, fallen skies lit air.

Near Oxford, by the stained canal
your latest love turned unkind. You
watched rainstorms fade. Wings burned banks blue.

When the drab days unwind you
do not put streams behind you.
Wait for the light to blind you.

Fade

Cliff Forshaw

A scene from *Fellini's Roma* fills my mind:
the crew are filming an archaeological dig.
It's all chiaroscuro underground:

arc-lights prod at dark; the judder of a klieg
as a wall gives way. Beyond light-rig, mic-boom,
this wormhole, ghosting faces, suddenly brightly archaic.

The crew have broken through to unmapped catacombs.
Light squints. The camera tracks the beam, catches
ancients almost stepping down from walls, zooms

to a shy face, surprised by the scrutiny of light.
The fresco shimmers, trembles – all this looks *live.*
    Do they smile?
Then paint disintegrates before your eyes.

What's killing them is us, our light, our atmosphere.
The chemistry we had is gone. They flee
from us and our machinery,

soak back into the airless soft volcanic rock.
We're lumbering slowly underground once more,
with tripods, meters, battery-packs:

all the impedimenta of our electric realm,
our hibernant or errant memories,
these brief revenants we've caught on film.

*

YouTube shows I'd got it wrong: a Roman villa's
unearthed by subway excavation for the impatient city;
the future's put on hold by the painted dead, old pillars.

What I'd remembered as serendipity
was pseudo-doc, mocked up, staged and lit. We see
the murals at first immured, before discovery.

Suspend yourself. You are the only lens.
They stare at you. Accuse. Then you are looking out
through painted eyes as the cutter's shiny glans

pokes through. And I'd forgotten much more:
those long perspectives of white-masked engineers;
the underground stream that echoes the helmets' tiny stars.

The frescoes fade, the faces evaporate,
and it's the stuff we breathe that makes them disappear.
We are left wading in an underground stream, torch-lit,

could be the Acheron or Styx.
The soundtrack howls, but the wind is just FX.
You're back, mind dark, forgetful in the cinema's pit;

beyond the screen all our machinery of recovery lies dead.

Six Kinds of Silence

Sue Hardy-Dawson

Quieter than fallen leaves
empty gardens are ghosts
where no child's been
windows dream of faces
& doors have forgotten
long goodbyes or widening
to welcome. The shades
of unwatched clouds hang
over vacant hills, staring
at roads – endlessly waiting.

Celebration

Sue Hardy-Dawson

The colour of night
is beautiful
expressionless and silent

though moon's face
seems empty
her still smile falls
like ribbon over the grey cherry

a moth's gaze
finds a fool's silver
under glass

beyond darkness
a cat's laughter
travels with the wind.

Between the Covers

A.F. Harrold

I sit soft on the sofa
with snow whipping my eyes,
with chill rock against my cheek.

Wolves howl,
but their tiny voices
vanish in the storm.

I need shelter,
to get under cover,
find a cave.

My cloak so thin,
my boots full of slush,
my eyes sting and my cheeks crackle.

I get up,
make a cup of tea,
look out the kitchen window at the summer.

A blackbird hops on the fence,
eying worms,
singing his snatch of sunlit song,

and then –
back to the sofa,
back to the mountain,
back to the winter,
back to the book.

Three Childhood Smells

A.F. Harrold

i.

It's a Friday night, probably in November.
Outside fog dandelions orange streetlights,
while indoors steam from a hot run bath
billows onto the landing, fogs the windows.

Downstairs *Roseanne's* laugh track roars,
and the rolling floral wave of bubble bath
wraps like an extra layer of dressing gown,
seeps comfort all through the little house.

Later, your passed on water's warm but dull.
This grey washed up soup of dead bubbles,
no matter how much hot I thunder in,
remains unfoamable, sudless, secondhand.

ii.

A vinegar fishhook at the backdoor's creak.
It's Tuesday night and you're finally home.
Dad's had plates warming for ten minutes.
Cutlery's been sat on the side, ready for this.

It's *Fastnet Fisheries* who've given us this gift,
wrapped in layers of thick, grease-spotted paper.
Each portion's opened, peered at, named,
and placed onto a plate. Steam pours up.

Ketchup's banged out. Cats caw circles like gulls.
Extra salt's shaken. Every week it's the same:
you stop off, pick up this battered bounty,
coming home from your weekly weighing in.

iii.

The white milk glug of calamine lotion.
The brown bottle uptips and cotton wool
dabs home the chalky smell, a scent-cuddle.
I'm back on the sofa, tiny, off-school and sick.

Someone comes back from the corner shop
with the other bottle only bought for the ill,
that sparkling elixir, sharp and sticky and queer,
the energised yellow-orange cure-all, Lucozade.

We had one blanket, just for the rare sick days,
soft embroidered with a rabbit and his carrot.
It made a sofa a sickbed, a place of doctoring.
(I saw it years later. Startled how small it was.)

The Moth & The New Moon

A.F. Harrold

The paper globe rattles, rustles and falls silent.

This is my study. This is late in the evening.

I look at the me looking back at me from the window.
From behind him endless blackness looks in on both of us.

The lampshade bursts back into brief life.
Dry paper shaking. A black-grey flutter inside.

I wonder how moths were before the lightbulb.

How did they feel unable to get to their goal,
the old bright moon untouched in orbit?

Is life more fulfilling these days, these nights
when the light's within their wingbeats' reach?

No moth knew this stark white warmth before.

The paper ball rattles, rustles and falls silent.

Mrs de Wilting

Lynne Reid Banks

It's too, too sweet of you dear things
To ask me to address you,
And tell you all about myself.
I hope it won't depress you
If I tell you all the details
Of my latest operation –
Done long before the lockdown,
But I'm still in isolation.
I've got a truly awful scar,
Though not where I can show it.
My mother told me men are brutes,
And now, my dears, I know it!
But now is surely not the time
To speak of ugly things,
When life can be so beautiful
If you keep your soul on wings!
Souls? God's a puzzle, don't you find?
One would so like to know
How he could make such strange mistakes!
Those plates – the ones below
That hold the world together.
You'd think he'd make them fit,
To stop the earthquakes, and those waves!
But not a bit of it.
And now we're covid stricken
Some punishment, perhaps?
For over-population?
Or is it some godly lapse?
My son's got religion.

He says God's not to blame.
It's Nature, and it would be bad
If Nature were too tame.
Disasters give us such a chance
To practice our compassion!
And to prevent the media
Being nothing else but fashion!
With lockdown, who cares what one wears?
I've not dressed up for weeks!
I only wish the Cabinet
Weren't such a bunch of geeks!
Why can't they give some clear advice?
It's really hardly fair
That in this crisis, our PM
Can't even brush his hair.
My husband's making faces.
I've not told you half my views!
But I can't stand more than an hour
In my lovely Gucchi shoes.
So thank you all for listening.
I hope we meet again.
If you should need a speaker
For a suitable campaign,
One I can give my 'yes' to –
I hope you'll think of me –
I'll come as soon as ever
I can get my PPE!

Lenten Lockdown

Paul Matthews

I gaze first thing out over rooftops
and let any lingering dreams
resolve in the mist above the river.

A low ridge marks the flight path
into Gatwick, but since lockdown
no jet trails veil the horizon.

Friends deliver bread to our door;
primroses everywhere. How then
to delight in it when so many are

gasping for air as the day breaks?
We must stand two metres apart.
If any dream lingers, let love fill
the distance between.

Faded Rainbows

Marcus Christopherson

Empty streets,
Faded rainbows,
Faintest hope
Stuck on windows.

Mouths covered,
Earth stood still,
Curtains twitch
Above the sill.

Times are strange
But people stronger.
Stay alert
In times of sonder.

Life is precious,
Moments more.
We keep on going
Behind closed doors.

Lockdown – a tribute to Adlestrop

Trevor Millum

Yes, I remember Lockdown,
The name, because one season of sun
The village was placed there
Unwontedly. Too late for anyone

To flee. Someone cleared their throat –
No one approached. No one came
Except delivery men and women.
What I recall was Lockdown, the name

And cherry blossom and forget-me-nots,
Honeysuckle and honesty,
No whit less lucid white and lovely
Than the high cloudlets in the sky.

And at that time, a blackbird sang
Close by, and round him, lustier,
Farther and farther, all the birds
Of Yorkshire and Lincolnshire.

My outlet in times of trouble

Mark Andrew Heathcote

Natures my outlet in times of trouble
When I want to get away from the news,
that COVID-19 self-isolation bubble,
rivers and long canal walks lift my blues.
They're an artery to a heartland,
only a soul's inner peace can understand.

It's my outlet when I see those gowns-of-white
gloved-and-masked - taking on-the-task
of saving lives, walking avenues of lime-
trees in a mindful and elegiac-
stride, writing some blank verse from time to time,
as I ponder how nature is sublime

It's surreal all the changes we've had,
all that's now forbidden, we took-for-granted
but truly in-other ways, I'm just-glad
holding one dear hand in mine supplanted
knowing-really nothing is-decided
however, the future gets lopsided.

It's in our grasp to hold this stinging-nettle
dull its sting by admiring everything,
it's in our courage, our hearts-metal
to fight fatigue tooth-and-nail with every limb,
recalling all that's perished before us
Once more rises in spring beauteous.

Lockdown & My Chai

Ashish Kapoor

It wasn't too long, I think about a month ago
I was at Starbucks, waiting for my chai to-go
Oh! The aroma at the cafe; I can still feel that taste
Oh! I miss them all, yummy cheese and carrot cake

'Chai tea latte for Ash', I want to hear once more
But it's Covid lockdown, am not going out for sure
Need a solution faster, how can I start my day
Hey, if there's no Sunshine, how can I make hay?

Combinations and permutations, all of them I tried
I want that same taste, it was quite loud that I cried
Suddenly, the weather changed with thunder and light
Gods could see, I wanted my chai, I was ready to fight

Then lightning struck my door, as if they casted a spell
Gods were up to something, was I being sent to hell?
I think it's just a warning. Or is it over, am dead?
Or maybe it's just the lockdown playing with my head.

Not Just Writer

Rita Rana

They call it pen, I call it magical wand
they call it paper, I call it canvas
they call it vocabulary, I call it emotions
they call it literature, I call it art
For them poetry is just rhyming, for me poetry is musical
flow of feelings,
for them a story is just an imagination, for me a story
is someone' s reality
for them essays are just an opinion, for me essays are
someone's experiences
for them writing is just a literary work, for me writing
is an adventurous and beautiful journey,
for them books are just a combination of pages and words
for me books are all aspects of life
for them writers are just a writer
for me writers are creators of living thoughts.

First the dust

Ariadne Radi Cor

I cannot write if there is dust around the desk, so I start hoovering the studio early, and while I am there, I hoover the rest of the house. I am done by 9 AM, but by then a line of light illuminates a thousand white atoms of dust drifting in mid-air, hovering from room to room, following my steps. I hit a cushion and the air in the room comes alive with soaring atoms. Since I cannot write with all these atoms around, I take the cushions out and slap them thoroughly with a carpet beater. The effort makes me cry, so I rest for a moment by the front door, and notice that the flowers on the porch are dying. I go back in and look for a jug to water them. It is 9:30 AM, the time I should start writing. Flowers first, writing second. The sink is full of dishes and the jug will not fit under the tap unless I wash up first. Jug first, flowers second. I cannot help noticing the atoms of grime lodged at the back of the sink. I cannot write if there is decay around me. Decay first, dishes second. As I scrape the old limescale off, my nails break. I cannot type with a broken nail, so I look for a nail filer in the bathroom upstairs. As I rummage in the drawer, I see a woman in the mirror. She looks flustered in her green pinafore, and her eyes are swollen. She tells me something about how the dust lives in the air, and we cannot get rid of the air or we will die, because the dust keeps us alive and gives us purpose. Back downstairs, I sit in the living room and pair my broken nails, my protruding bones—what should I wear, and does it even matter anymore? I conclude that I cannot write the eulogy in all this dust. It is 11 AM, so I thaw the frozen canapes—how many people will actually come, ten?—and start worrying about where I should arrange the urn, but first, the wake, then the urn. First the nails, then the canapes. First the decay, then the flowers and the cushions.

Gravity Ungrateful

Mark Blickley

Gravity Ungrateful
Yes, I am dressed in mourning
Dark clothes for a dark time
Yet I yearn to escape
Pandemic imprisonment
With the germ of an idea
That will allow me to soar
Above my confinement
In an airborne threat
Against complacency and boredom
As I reach up to a blue heaven
That promises social distancing
On a cosmic scale,
But that old bitch gravity
Bears down on me,
Slapping me down
Like a petulant child
Crying out
For what she cannot have,
Slammed back
To a blanketed earth
Of red white and blue.

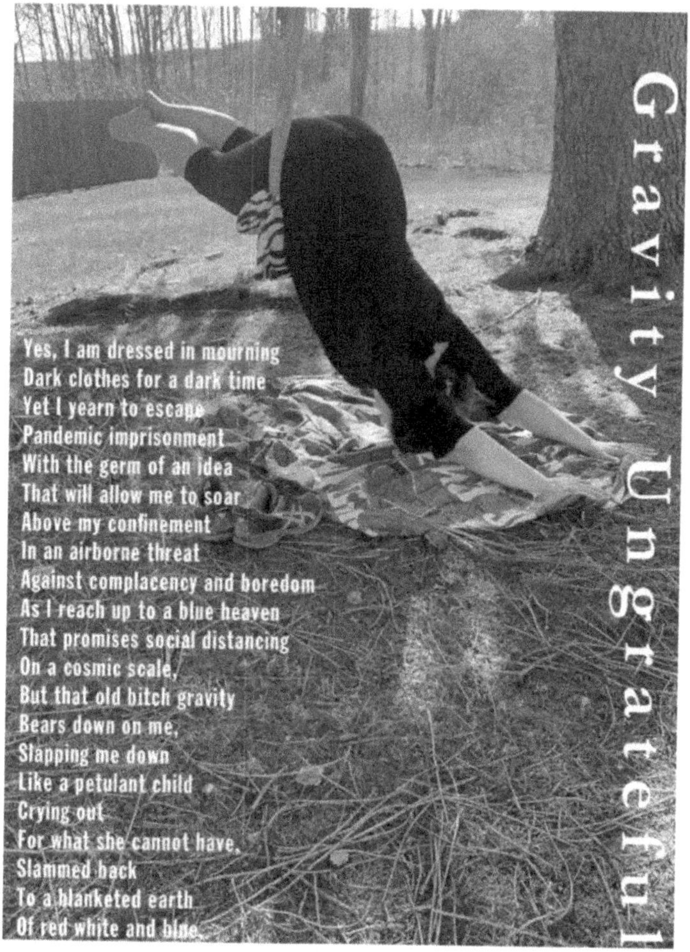

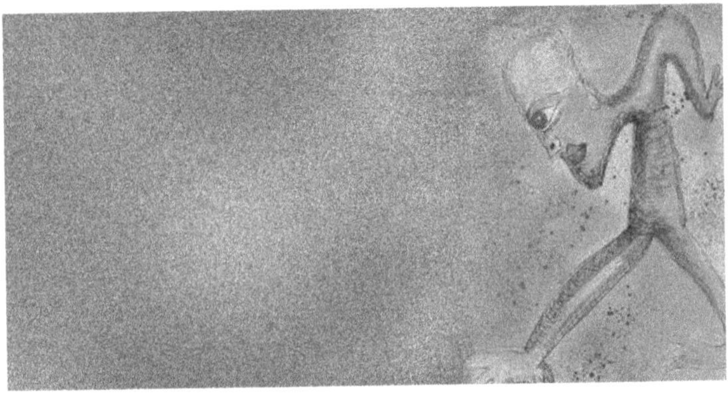

An Evening Walk

Francis H Powell

A landscape opens out
Different shades of green
all to absorb
as branches fill out
with shouts of spring
There is almost deafening
sound of silence
just the repetitive strains
of my dog panting
as he pulls one way then another
tracking some indecipherable scent
as birds make distant calls
chattering in far off trees
messages both confusing and bold
The sky is melancholic
with a sad message to tell
I pass through the carpet of green
and arrive back amongst houses

that look as dead as sleeping giants
Oh look up there, I spot a light on
perhaps a parent reading a child
a bed time story, a precious moment
drawing a line under the day
A parent's duties complete
I am nearly home, more signs of life
But as we all know we are all know
we are shut in, and my walk was a brief
moment of freedom.

Insides Longing For Outsides

Sally Kindberg

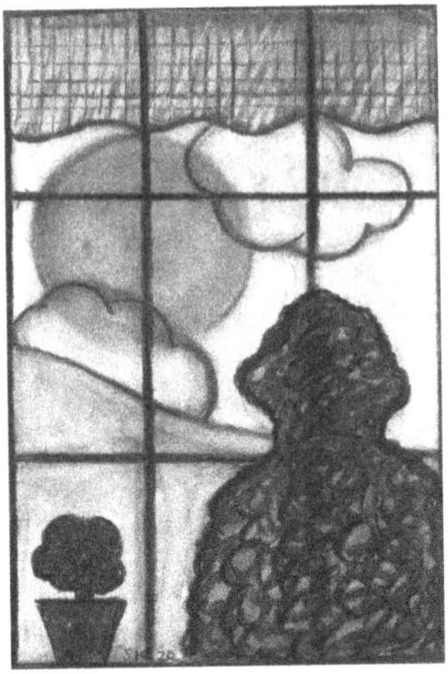

Me in a cube in a rectangle

Sally Kindberg

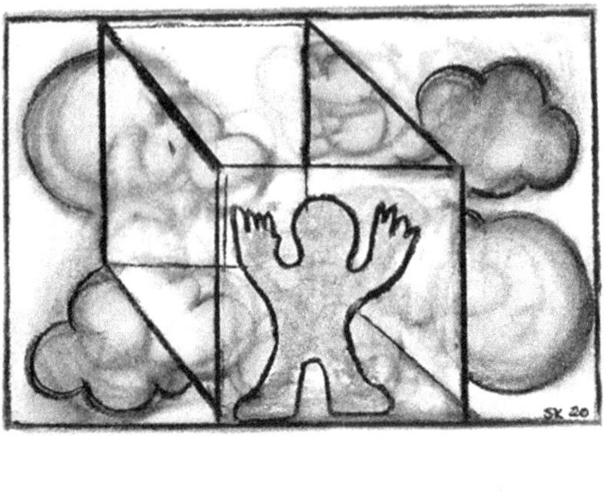

Pairidaeza Scrolldown

Paula Claire

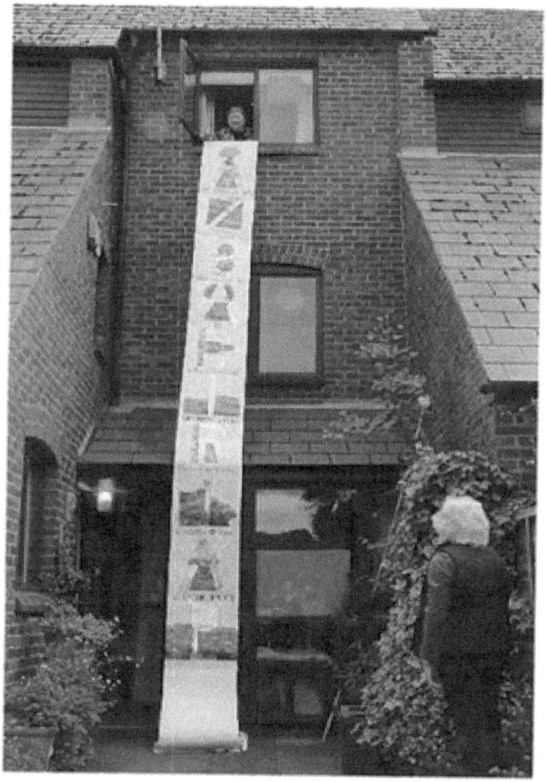

A visual poem celebrating our Residents' Association tradition of Gardens Open Day, in 2020 restricted by Lockdown

The 22-foot-long paper scrolldown was displayed 3-4pm Saturday 20 May, Oxford. People gathered to say the lines conducted by Paula from her window, then welcome to visit the garden to see the scroll more closely, observing the current rule: no more than 6 together.

'PAIRIDAEZA' is an ancient Persian word, at first meaning 'an enclosed place;' then it extended to mean 'a walled orchard;' later flowers were grown there, becoming 'a garden;' finally this Persian garden form developed with a cross of water channels and fountains becoming an emblem of the Heavenly Garden: PARADISE.

We live in Paradise, the name of the site of the gardens of the medieval Friaries outside Westgate/Southgate, their lands stretching down to the fertile alluvial soils by the Thames, Our houses are a redevelopment from the demolished Victorian gasworks slums; our walled gardens tiny but each one characterful, a refuge during this unprecedented period of Lockdown.

My poem created on wallpaper lining has 10 sections, 1 for each of the 10 capital letters of PAIRIDAEZA. I have appliqued gold paper for the letters and decorated them with cut-outs of garden photos from flower catalogues and Country Life magazine. Between each letter is a line. Reading from the bottom upwards – traditionally Earth to Heaven, the handwritten poem lines say:

1. An enclosed place
2. A walled orchard
3. Flowers become a garden
4. Lockdown in our gardens
5. on ancient Friary ground
6. "You are NOT confined…
7. Observe and Consider" – advice from the enclosed Order, the Poor Clares of Arundel who have chosen permanent Lockdown as a way of life.
8. Kingfishers dart our Stream again – seen again after some years' absence.

9. LOST PARADISE FOUND – let us hope the quiet and clean air of Lockdown will be as far as possible maintained in 'the new normal,' showing proper respect for our environment and beneficial to all aspects of our health.

Featured on the back cover:
PAIRIDAEZA SCROLLDOWN visual poem for lockdown by PoetArtist Paula Claire, Oxford 20 June 2020. Photo ©Paul San Casciani. Paula Claire at 2nd floor window having let down her poem guided by a neighbour.

Credits

Image and photograph credits:

Quentin Blake, p.152, illustration reproduced with the permission of United Agents on behalf of Quentin Blake.

Paula Claire, p.307 + back cover (Photo ©Paul San Casciani).

Brook Fischer, p.78.

Annabel Fitch, p.81

Beatrice Georgalidis, photograph p.303.

John Hegley, p.17.

Josh Hudes, p.105, 180.

Robin Hulbert-Powell, p.76.

Stephanie Hulbert-Powell, p.45, 46, 106.

Sally Kindberg, p.306.

David Melling, p.149.

Francis H Powell, p.38, 49, 51, 75, 86, 109, 113, 143, 145, 150, 171, 177, 182, 201, 212, 213, 221, 254, 277, 304

Mukul Samaria, p.261.

James Sheppard, images for themes *Funny stuff in Lockdown, Time in Lockdown.*

Arthur Smith, p.19.

Olga Solabarrieta, images for themes *Deep Thoughts, Children in Lockdown, Love in Lockdown, Hope and Despair, Loneliness and Emptiness, Land and Sea, Different Perspectives, p.79*

Monique Tell, p.204.

Andy J Tyler, p.186, 230.

Barnabas Wetton, p.37.

Chris White, p.104.

Other credits:

Katrina Naomi, *Wild Persistence*, Seren, 2020

Grace from *A Portable Paradise* (Peepal Tree Press, 2019) reproduced by kind permission of Peepal Tree Press.